Contributors

Neil Armstrong
Head of Postgraduate School of Medicine and Health Sciences, University of Exeter

Jenny Bell
Research Fellow and Clinical Exercise Practitioner, British Association for Cardiac Rehabilitation, Ketton, Stamford, Lincolnshire

Richard Budgett
Chief Medical Officer British Olympic Association and British Olympic Medical Centre, Northwick Park Hospital, Harrow, Middlesex

Andrew Clark
Senior Lecturer and Honorary Consultant Cardiologist, Castle Hill Hospital, University of Hull

Christopher Clark
Consultant Physician, Hairmyres Hospital, East Kilbride

Lorna Cochrane
Staff Grade in Respiratory Medicine, Hairmyres Hospital, East Kilbride

Yvette Cooper
Public Health Minister, Department of Health

Susie Dinan
Research Fellow and Clinical Exercise Practitioner, The Royal Free Hospital and University College School of Medicine, London

Michael Doherty
Professor of Rheumatology, University of Nottingham Medical School

John Etherington
Consultant in Rheumatology and Rehabilitation, Defence Services Medical Rehabilitation Centre, Headley Court, Epsom, Surrey

Mairi Gould
Research Fellow, Department of Primary Care and Population Sciences, Royal Free and University College Medical School, London

Mark Harries
Consultant Physician, Department of Respiratory Medicine, Northwick Park Hospital, Harrow, Middlesex

Steve Iliffe
Reader in General Practices, Department of Primary Care and Population Sciences, Royal Free and University College Medical School, London

Bob Laventure
British Heart Foundation, National Centre for Physical Activity and Health, Loughborough University

Donald Macleod
Consultant General Surgeon, St John's Hospital, Howden, Livingstone, West Lothian

Simon Mockett
Lecturer, Division of Physiotherapy Education, University of Nottingham

Sharon See Tai
Operational Research Analyst, Department of Primary Care and Population Sciences, Royal Free and University College Medical School, London

Patrick Sharp
Consultant Physician, Department of Diabetes and Endocrinology, Northwick Park Hospital, Harrow, Middlesex

Paul Smith
Research Fellow, Department of Primary Care and Population Sciences, Royal Free and University College Medical School, London

David Sword
Senior House Officer in Respiratory Medicine, Hairmyres Hospital, East Kilbride

Nick Webborn
Medical Adviser to the National Sports Medicine Institute, c/o Medical College of St Bartholomew's Hospital, London

Archie Young
Professor of Geriatric Medicine, Department of Clinical and Surgical Sciences, University of Edinburgh

Editors' introduction

In the ten years since The Royal College of Physicians published the report *Medical Aspects of Exercise; Benefits and Risks* (London: RCP, 1991), the body of evidence for the benefits of exercise has continued to grow and to be refined. In addition, our attitude to the risks of exercise has matured. No longer does the underlying philosophy emphasise the exclusion of those at increased risk of adverse events. Indeed, it is currently recognised that these are often the very people who have most to gain by increasing their habitual level of physical activity. The emphasis now is on enabling each individual's safe and effective participation, taking due account of their particular vulnerabilities. This fundamental change in approach owes much to the growing number of exercise instructors who are experienced in guiding and supervising specific groups of patients, often building on models of practice developed in cardiac rehabilitation. The programme for the conference upon which this publication is based reflected these developments.

The conference explored why and how doctors might incorporate an appropriate exercise prescription into the management of their patients. It was not possible in the time available to cover all the disease states where exercise can make an important contribution. Nor was it possible to give an exhaustive account of both the evidence base and the practicalities of delivery for each of the clinical conditions or situations that were included. Instead, we concentrated on examples that would illustrate the range and magnitude of the therapeutic opportunities and the principles underpinning their safe and effective implementation for those who need them most.

Chapters 1–5 concentrate on the evidence for benefit and on the underlying physiology in five selected areas. Chapters 6–12 then concentrate on some of the practicalities of enabling safe and effective exercise participation in a further seven types of practice. Finally, chapters 13–15 look to the future and to the professional, training and political developments, which seem likely to support our efforts to use exercise effectively for the benefit of our patients.

ARCHIE YOUNG
MARK HARRIES
May 2001

Contents

THE FUTURE:

THE OLIVER-SHARPEY LECTURE

1 The health benefits of physical activity for patients recovering from injury

John Etherington

Introduction

The military medical services have extensive experience of the management of musculo-skeletal injury. The burden of such injuries in the military is high; between 35–45% of all general practice attendances in the services are related to musculo-skeletal conditions. In a prospective study of 2,000 male army recruits during basic training 43.9% sustained an injury and 44.6% of those injured had a second or further injury.[1]

The Armed Forces are concerned to reduce the morbidity of these injuries to the individual, the cost of treatment and the loss of operational effectiveness through reduced manpower. Within the Army alone 70% of the working days lost to ill health are due to musculo-skeletal disease. But the burden of musculo-skeletal disease is not confined to the military. There is a 40% 12-month period prevalence and an 80% lifetime prevalence of low back pain within the general population, and musculo skeletal disease is the commonest cause of disability and working days lost in the civilian population.

Reducing the burden of musculo-skeletal injury

The cost and morbidity of injury may be reduced by measures such as the introduction of safety mechanisms and the eradication of foul play in sport. In the workplace injury prevention may depend on the development of methods of predicting those at highest risk of injury[1] and developing specific preventive measures. This approach may be possible in a closely constrained environment such as an army training regiment but not necessarily for the general population. There, the aim is to improve the general level of exercise and conditioning to prevent musculo-skeletal injury or ameliorate pain caused by injury.

Exercise-based rehabilitation

Exercise has a role in the treatment of established injury. The original exponents of this form of treatment, and currently the organisation most

1

involved in its prescription, are the Defence Medical Services. Military rehabilitation was not developed from evidence-based medicine. It is a pragmatically designed model based on the treatment of mass casualties and aims to provide the quickest path to health for the maximal number of patients using the minimum of staff.

The Defence Services Medical Rehabilitation Centre is based at Headley Court near Epsom and uses this principle to treat in excess of 2,000 in-patients per year. Back pain cases constitute the largest proportion of those treated at Headley Court (41.5%), followed by knee injuries (20.5%). However, numerous other musculo-skeletal conditions are treated and there is a small neurological rehabilitation unit. A proportion of those rehabilitating will return to Headley Court for final conditioning to levels of fitness compatible with return to the more demanding roles in the Armed Forces (eg in the infantry).

Military rehabilitation involves the use of group therapy, which consists of a graded programme of exercise delivered to 12–20 patients grouped by region of injury and their level of function. They have a fully programmed day of 10 half hour sessions during which time they will be exercising. A remedial instructor (a military exercise therapist) directs them through a programme of rehabilitation lasting up to four weeks. This role (previously undertaken by the remedial gymnast) is fulfilled by a trained physical training instructor, who has completed a seven-month course in anatomy, physiology and in the principles of exercise-based rehabilitation. Remedial instructors are the linch-pin of the programme. Patients enter the groups, receive their treatment and are then discharged back to work, where they are directed to continue their own specifically prescribed programme. They may return later to Headley Court for further rehabilitation in either the same group, or if they have progressed, at a higher level of functional activity. Additional therapy such as physiotherapy, occupational therapy, social work and speech and language therapy are available and patients are programmed for these as appropriate. It is made clear to the patient that these are not the main elements of their rehabilitation, but that they complement the exercise-based therapy. Likewise medical input, although consultant led, is kept to a minimum to allow the patients to return to an expectation of health and reduce their reliance on medical support.

Military rehabilitation relies on military ethos, compliance with treatment, competitiveness within the group and the skills of the remedial instructor. Fundamentally, it relies on exercise physiology to modify the effects of musculo-skeletal injury. The programme for rehabilitation includes increasing the joint range of movement, development of local muscular endurance followed by muscular strength and then power if it is appropriate for the individual's occupation. Throughout, there is work designed to maintain and develop aerobic capacity.

Psychological re-training is also important within the programme and involves education of the individual as to the nature of the injury they have sustained and the process by which it will recover. It is necessary to re-introduce the individual back to the social ethos with which they are familiar and this involves the re-introduction of elements of work and recreation. Patients are given administrative and managerial duties, expected to attend unit social occasions and are returned to formal group exercise. Exercise is perceived as an element of daily work within the military and to be exercising within a group is therefore considered as a return to work, important when injury may have isolated the individual from their operational unit. There is an attempt to 'empower' the individual by giving both directed time for rehabilitation and undirected time during which they must decide which elements of the rehabilitation programme they will pursue. Nevertheless, a large element of the musculo-skeletal rehabilitation in military relies on 'disempowerment' and the acceptance that compliance will occur in most circumstances.

Outcomes in military rehabilitation

Does the programme work? The main outcome of interest in military rehabilitation is return to work. There is a system of medical grading, which allows us to judge whether a patient can return back to full duties or in a restricted capacity. Of 206 patients with mechanical low back pain, 29.6% increased their medical category during admission, with 20% returned to be fit for all duties. Approximately 14% of low back pain patients lost function, as measured by medical grading. For some of these patients, this was due to a true loss in functional capacity but in many cases the reduced medical grading was due to an appropriate grading being given to an individual for the first time. Outcomes appear better in other groups of patients, eg those rehabilitating after anterior cruciate ligament (ACL) reconstruction in which 38% gain in medical occupational grading and 31% are fit for all duties after admission.

There was a low rate of medical discharge from the Armed Forces: 2.4% in the mechanical low back pain group and 2.3% in the ACL group. Therefore, in excess of 97% of the mechanical low back pain patients will still be employed within the services in some capacity. This is much higher than the rate of return to work in people with chronic low back pain in civilian practice. This probably reflects the capacity to provide a relatively sheltered working environment and the fact that patients have remained in a working environment throughout the course of their injury and rehabilitation. Maintaining the expectation of productive work appears to be very important in terms of producing a good occupational outcome.

Not all types of injury respond as well to exercise-based rehabilitation, for example patella fractures. Only 13% of the patients improve their occupational medical grading and a similar proportion experience a reduction, with a higher rate of medical discharge, 3.4%. The reasons why exercise based rehabilitation fails in some contexts may be illustrated by a study performed by Carter *et al.*[3] This study of the rehabilitation of ACL injuries showed significant improvements in measures of muscular strength and overall function after a four week period. However, joint position sense did not improve significantly. This may indicate that there are elements of an injury that are not directly affected by the patterns of exercise being used.

Evidence for benefit of exercise in rehabilitation

There is a lack of good quality randomised controlled trials of therapy and rehabilitation after injury. A recent systematic review commissioned by the Ministry of Defence from the Cochrane musculo-skeletal Injuries Group examined interventions after exercise related injury.[4] It found a paucity of good quality clinical trials. Only five recommendations could be made for treatment strategies showing clear evidence of benefit, only one of which related to exercise-based rehabilitation. This was the use of functional bracing in the rehabilitation of tibial stress fractures and even this conclusion was based on limited and questionable data.

There is evidence for the benefit of exercise in low back pain. One of the best studies to support the use of exercise-based rehabilitation in low back pain was a single blind randomised controlled trial carried out by the Oxford group with a two-year follow-up after intervention.[5,6] This showed a 7.7% reduction in the Oswestry Low Back Pain Disability Index compared with only 2.4% fall in the control group.

Most recently there has been a Cochrane library review of exercise therapy for low back pain.[7] Thirty nine randomised controlled trials were identified. There was strong evidence that exercise therapy was no more effective than other active or inactive treatments for acute low back pain. There was conflicting evidence for exercise in chronic low back pain when compared with inactive treatments, but exercise therapy was more effective than the usual care delivered by the general practitioner and as effective as conventional physiotherapy. There was no evidence as to which exercises were more effective than others but there may have been some evidence that combination programmes including elements of exercise, physiotherapy, occupational therapy and back school may have better outcomes than single modality therapies.

Why is there such limited evidence of benefit? Does it indicate that exercise is truly ineffective in the treatment of musculo-skeletal injury or are we underestimating its effect? Many studies were excluded from the Cochrane review because of poor design and generally their outcome measures lacked sensitivity. Furthermore, the subjective benefits of exercise are difficult to assess. Studies designed to examine conditions considered to be single disease entities, such as back pain, are really observing a collection of heterogeneous conditions frequently treated by a variety of heterogeneous modalities.

Conclusion

Exercise appears to be beneficial in rehabilitation after injury and this may be mediated by a variety of factors including pain reduction either by distraction or centrally operating endorphin mechanisms. There is clearly a physiological response from bone, muscle and the immune system which would aid recovery after injury, and there are major psychological benefits, not least the return of function and return to society in a group setting with people with similar injuries.

Physical activity after injury is based on sound physiological principles but there is limited evidence available to support its clinical use. The challenge for the future is to provide robust evidence for the role of exercise in rehabilitation after injury and in particular to identify those modalities of treatment which are the most effective, and the sub-groups of disease and injury in which the benefits are greatest. The principles of exercise-based rehabilitation are applicable at all levels of physical activity and the benefits may be greatest where people are most unfit. It is an approach to therapy that should be considered for use within the general population and not just the military.

References

1   Etherington J, Johnston B, Owen G, et al. Prediction of musculo-skeletal injury in military recruits using artificial neural networks. *Rheumatology Oxford* 2000; **39**(Abstracts suppl. 1): 124.

2   Campbell H, O'Driscoll S. The epidemiology of leisure accidents in Scotland. *Health Bull* 1995; **53**: 280–93.

3   Carter ND, Jenkinson TR, Wilson D, et al. Joint position sense and rehabilitation in the anterior cruciate ligament deficient knee. *Br J Sports Med* 1997; **31**: 209–12.

4 Gillespie WJ, Quinn KM, Handoll HHG. *Research Study on the Effectiveness of Interventions to Prevent or Treat Musculoskeletal Injuries in Soldiers.* Report to the Ministry of Defence,1997.

5 Frost H, Klaber Moffett JA, Moser JS, Fairbank JC. Randomised controlled trial for evaluation of fitness programme for patients with chronic low back pain. *Br Med J* 1995; **310**: 151–4.

6 Frost H, Lamb SE, Klaber Moffett JA, *et al.* A fitness programme for patients with chronic low back pain: 2-year follow-up of a randomised controlled trial. *Pain* 1998; **75**: 273–9.

7 Tulder MW van, Malmivaara A, Esmail R, Koes B. *Exercise Therapy for Low Back Pain. (Cochrane Review).* The Cochrane Library. Issue 3. Oxford: Update Software, 2000.

2 | The health benefits of physical activity for patients with osteoarthritis

Simon Mockett and Michael Doherty

The nature of OA

Osteoarthritis (OA) is by far the commonest form of joint disorder. Although it may affect any synovial joint, it selectively targets knees, hips and certain small joints (finger distal interphalangeal joints, thumb base, great toe metatarsophalangeal joint, cervical and lumbar facet joints). OA is a major cause of locomotor pain, the single most important cause of disability and handicap from arthritis, and an important community health care burden. It shows a strong association with ageing. With the increasing 'greying' of the population, large joint OA, especially of the knee, will become an even more important health care challenge.

OA is commonly viewed as a degenerative 'wear and tear' disease, the inevitable consequence of ageing, that always progresses despite medical interventions, and about which nothing definitive can be done other than total joint replacement. Over the last decade, however, this pessimistic view of OA has changed as we have learned more about its pathophysiology and epidemiology. The following observations particularly deserve emphasis:

- OA has accompanied man throughout evolutionary history and a similar process occurs in other animals with synovial joints
- the distribution of joint involvement in OA, which differs between animals, remains unexplained but joints which are targeted by OA are those that have greatly changed in recent evolution and which may not have fully adapted to their new functions and thus have little mechanical reserve
- most structural OA in the community, determined by joint examination or X-rays, does not cause symptoms or functional impairment. This is particularly true of small joint involvement
- symptoms that associate with OA are most often episodic rather than persistent, and often improve. The natural history of symptomatic OA of hands, knees or hips is not necessarily progressive and varies according to joint site

▌ although focal thinning and loss of articular hyaline cartilage is one of the cardinal pathological characteristics of OA (Fig 1), cartilage cells in an OA joint show increased metabolic activity, increased division and increased production of cartilage matrix components. The adjacent bone also shows increased activity and remodelling; at the joint margins there is production of new fibrocartilage that undergoes secondary endochondral ossification to form 'osteophytes', thus increasing the surface area of contact for the joint. The synovium undergoes hyperplasia often with limited metaplasia to osteochondral 'loose' bodies. The outer capsule also thickens and contracts, as if to maintain stability of the remodelling joint. In OA therefore all the tissues in the joint are displaying increased metabolic activity, producing new material, and remodelling the shape of the joint to better allow force transmission across it.

Such observations support the proposition that OA is the inherent repair process of synovial joints (Fig 2). A wide variety of joint insults may trigger this repair process. All the tissues of the joint depend on each other for normal function and health, therefore, insult to any individual component (cartilage, bone, synovium, ligament, muscle, nerve) will

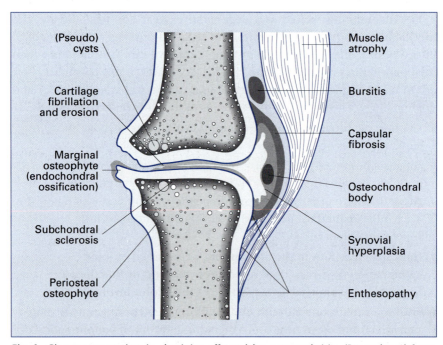

Fig 1. Changes occurring in the joint affected by osteoarthritis. (Reproduced from ref [1] with permission).

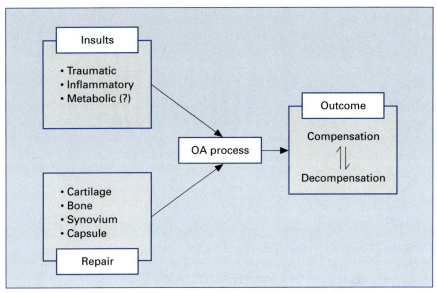

Fig 2. Diagrammatic representation of OA as the inherent repair process of synovial joints. (Reproduced from ref [1] with permission).

impact on the other tissues and lead to a similar OA phenotype. Sometimes we recognise the insult, such as major injury or a torn meniscus or ligament, but it is suggested the insults often remain unrecognised. Once triggered, however, all the joint tissues take part in this slow repair process. Often the repair compensates for the insult, resulting in an anatomically altered joint but one that does not associate with pain or disability, 'compensated OA'. In some cases, however, either because of overwhelming or chronic insult or a compromised sub-optimal repair response, repair cannot keep pace with the damage and the joint continues to lose tissue and more commonly associates with symptoms and disability, 'decompensated OA' or 'joint failure'.

Joint usage and OA

Joints are designed to move and all the tissues depend on regular movement, stretching or impact loading for maintained health and function (Fig 3). If a synovial joint is immobilised, all the tissues atrophy. At the other extreme, excessive or repeated mechanical overloading of a joint may result in tissue injury and joint damage. For example, repetitive occupational knee bending while carrying loads[2] or the excessive activity undertaken by some elite athletes[3,4] are risk factors for development of knee OA. It is somewhere between these two extremes of usage that

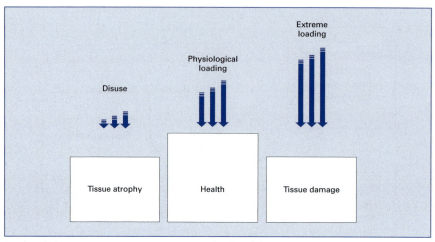

Fig 3. The relationship between loading and joint health is U-shaped not linear.

normal repetitive physiological loading and movement maintain the health of the normal joint. When a joint is compromised by OA it is at least as important that movement is maintained.

Pain, disability and OA

The correlations among pain, disability and structural X-ray changes of OA vary according to joint site. They are weak, if not absent, at small joints of the hand or spine and strongest at the hip. At the knee (Fig 4), there is good correlation between knee pain and disability but the correlations between these and structural change are only weak.[5] From various estimates,[6] the impact of knee pain, disability and structural (pathological) OA on a population of 100,000 older adults (aged ≥55 years) can be estimated as shown in Table 1 (data derived from ref [7]).

Correctable associations of knee pain, disability and OA

Better correlates with knee pain and disability than X-ray change are quadriceps weakness[5] psychological distress[8] lower formal education[9] and poor current health status.[8] Elements of these, unlike radiographic change, are potentially modifiable. Other local associations with knee OA that have been defined include reduced knee proprioception,[10] reduced standing balance[11] and increased lateral instability.[12] Apart from providing strength of movement, the quadriceps muscle is an important proprioceptive organ; weakness and reduced proprioception both may

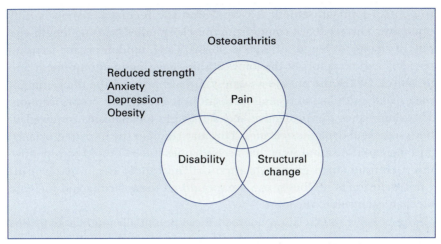

Fig 4. Pain and disability show only loose correlation with osteoarthritis structural change. Stronger correlations exist with the other, potentially modifiable, factors listed.

Table 1. Estimates of impact of knee pain, disability and structural (pathological) OA on a population of 100,000 older adults (aged ≥55 years) (derived from ref [7]).

Disability	N (out of 100,000)
Knee pain for at least 4 weeks in the last year	25,000
Knee pain and some disability	12,500
Knee pain, some disability and X-ray OA	7,500
Knee pain, severe disability and X-ray OA	1,500

contribute to impaired balance and abnormal gait. Obesity is a further strong risk factor for the development of knee pain, structural knee OA and more rapid radiographic progression. Losing weight, however, can improve knee pain and reduce the increased risk of further X-ray change.

Reduced muscle size, especially of the quadriceps, is a consistent feature of the knee OA and results in weakness. Also, full activation and recruitment of muscle fibres may be inhibited through spinal cord reflexes, pain inhibition or other mechanisms. This limits function in daily activities such as rising from sitting and climbing stairs. The OA patient may adapt by selectively self-limiting their activity. The subsequent reduction in joint movement may accentuate tissue atrophy and lead to further 'decompensation' of the OA process. Thus as the OA patient gets weaker, they get stiffer, more unfit and a downward spiral begins.

Muscles, however, have important functions other than strength. They are possibly the most important tissue for joint proprioception. In order to control joint movement it is vital that the feedback system is fully operative. This feedback comes from muscle spindles (sensing length and rate of change of length of muscle fibres), Golgi tendon organs (sensing tension) and receptors in the joint capsules (sensing joint movement and pressure). In OA the muscle weakness and atrophy and the thickening of the capsule, with loss of receptors, result in reduced joint proprioception. This diminishes the protective and stabilising mechanisms required in both static and dynamic activities. This may result in the impaired balance and increased postural sway that accompanies knee OA and to repetitive microtrauma through subtle inco-ordination of the moving joint ('microclutziness'). Obesity can compound all these factors and increase mechanical insult to the joint.

The possible interrelation between these potentially modifiable factors is outlined in Fig 5. It is clear that a change in one may result in changes in the others.

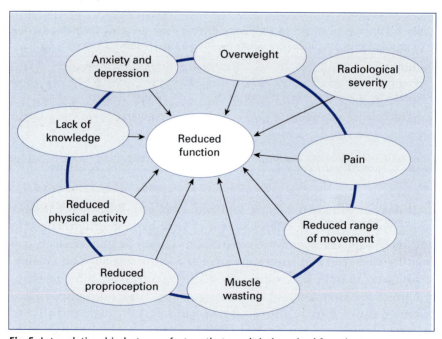

Fig 5. Interrelationship between factors that result in impaired function.

Exercise as an intervention for OA

A number of studies have examined the therapeutic efficacy of exercise in patients with large joint, predominantly knee, OA. These have differed in terms of patient age, type and intensity of exercise, duration of exercise supervision and length of follow-up. However, all concur in showing improvements with respect to pain and function, at least in the short term (up to 3–6 months). Furthermore exercise appears successful in a range of patients including the very elderly.

The results of a recent review of randomised clinical trials[13] are summarised in Table 2. The effect size is modest to good for both pain reduction and improvement in function (in general, an effect size of 0.2= a small beneficial effect, 0.5=a medium effect, and 0.8=a large effect). The study by Ettinger *et al* examined outcome over an 18-month period in 439 adults aged ≥60 years with knee OA.[14] In that study, there were two intervention arms, one employing aerobic fitness training and the other, progressive resistance strength training; both were compared to a group receiving only education about OA. Interestingly, both types of exercise gave beneficial, long-term results. Improvements from strengthening exercise could come from the demonstrated increase in strength and improvement in knee proprioception from such exercise[10,11] with possible secondary benefits from improved balance and co-ordination together with the possibility of contributing to weight control. Aerobic training improves well-being and increases the duration of restorative delta sleep, with possible benefits in terms of pain perception and severity. Most exercise programmes combine elements of both types of exercise, though it is unclear whether the benefits of each are additive.

All the studies in Table 2 involved supervised exercise, often in a group

Table 2. Best evidence synthesis.

First Author (reference)	Pain	Self-reported disability	Observed disability in walking
Acceptable validity, sufficient power			
Van Baar[15]	0.58 (0.54, 0.62)	0.26 (0.22, 0.30)	0.28 (0.24, 0.32)
Ettinger[14] (aerobic exercise)	0.47(0.44, 0.50)	0.41 (0.38, 0.44)	0.89 (0.85, 0.93)
Ettinger[14] (resistance exercise)	0.31 (0.28, 0.34)	0.36 (0.33, 0.39)	0.31 (0.28, 0.34)
Low validity or power			
Börjesson[16]	0.20 (0.08, 0.32)	NM	−0.11 (−0.17, −0.05)
Kovar[17]	0.52 (0.43, 0.61)	0.88 (0.78, 0.98)	0.92 (0.82, 1.02)

Values are effect sizes (95% confidence intervals) for each outcome measure.
NM = not measured.

class. Patients may derive mutual support from the group and thus have higher rates of adherence. This leads to reduced feelings of helplessness and depression and there is certainly more scope for patient education and reinforcement, which improve patients' ability to cope. But such interventions are expensive and time consuming.

A recent study by O'Reilly *et al*[18] of 191 community subjects with knee pain involved unsupervised strengthening exercise, including use of an elastic resistance band, after brief instruction and three subsequent contacts with a research nurse. Compared to a non-exercise control group such exercise gave improvements at six months follow-up in knee pain and lower limb function with concomitant increase in quadriceps strength.

Such simple and inexpensive intervention has now been applied in a larger randomised factorial trial of 786 community subjects with knee pain followed for two years (O'Reilly *et al*[19]). Over this longer period the home exercise subjects again showed benefits in terms of reduced pain, improved function and increased quadriceps strength. A clear dose-response effect was seen with respect to self-reported compliance (Table 3). It is salutary, but not surprising, that over half such subjects did not adhere to this suggested change in lifestyle over a two-year period. This is not dissimilar to experience with other chronic health interventions, be they pharmacological or non-pharmacological. Adherence to such an exercise programme will depend on multiple patient-centred factors such as their knowledge, beliefs and attitudes with respect to knee OA and its treatments; perceived benefits from other interventions; self-efficacy and 'willingness to change' their lifestyle. It should not be underestimated how difficult it might be for a patient to move through the 'stages of change'.[20] Such factors need to be addressed if any programme is to work effectively, particularly with respect to primary and secondary prevention of knee OA.

Additional benefits that may accrue from exercise, but for which there are few data for OA subjects, include:

Table 3. Effect of self-reported compliance over a two-year period.

Level of Compliance	N	Effect size for pain reduction at 2 years
Low	307	0.16
Medium	32	0.34
High	128	0.42

There is a dose response but many subjects did not adhere to the regimen.

∎ reduced tendency to fall. Exercise may reduce falls and fall-related injury in elderly subjects not specifically screened for OA,[21]

∎ reduction in obesity. Losing weight can reduce pain and disability from OA and possibly retard structural deterioration at the knee or hip.[22] Exercise plus conscious dieting appear more effective in reducing weight than either alone.

Exercise for primary prevention of OA

Primary prevention of decompensated, symptomatic OA is a matter of considerable importance but an area where we have few data. Theoretically, however, maintaining muscle power, proprioception, balance and co-ordination should delay or even prevent onset of symptoms and disability from OA in a large section of our ageing community.

Conclusion

There is strong theoretical and clinical trial evidence to support the prescription of both strengthening and aerobic exercise to patients with symptomatic large joint OA. This applies to patients of any age. Benefits may derive from the direct effects of exercise but there are also possible indirect gains, for example from reduction of obesity. There is also excellent face valdity for exercise as a central aspect of lifestyle modification in primary prevention of large joint OA.

The challenges for the future are to explain the exact physiological mechanisms by which exercise has its effects on the pathophysiological changes of OA, and to devise management strategies that patients are able to adhere to for long enough to effect a beneficial change in their lifestyle.

References

1   Doherty M. Osteoarthritis: new thoughts about an old disease, In: *Horizons in Medicine Vol 10*. London: Royal College of Physicians, 1998.

2   Felson DT, Hannan MT, Naimark A, *et al*. Occupational physical demands, knee bending and knee osteoarthritis: results from the Framingham Study. *J Rheumatol* 1991; **18**: 1587–92.

3   Kujala UM, Kaprio J, Sarna S. Osteoarthritis of weight bearing joints of lower limbs in former elite male athletes. *Br Med J* 1994; **308**: 231–4.

4   Kujala UM, Kettunen J, Paananen H, *et al*. Knee Osteoarthritis in Former Runners, Soccer players, Weight Lifters, and Shooters. *Arthritis Rheum* 1995; **38**: 539–46.

5   O'Reilly S, Jones A, Muir KR, Doherty M. Quadriceps weakness in knee osteoarthritis: the effect on pain and disability. *Ann Rheum Dis* 1998; **57**: 588–94.

6 Tennant A, Fear J, Pickering A, *et al.* Prevalence of knee problems in the population aged 55 and over: identifying the need for arthroplasty. *Br Med J* 1995; **310**: 1291–3.

7 Peat G, McCarney R, Croft P. Knee pain and osteoarthritis in older adults: a review of community burden and current use of primary health care. *Ann Rheum Dis* 2001; **60**: 91–7.

8 O'Reilly S, Muir KR, Doherty M. Knee pain and disability in the Nottingham community: association with poor health status and psychological distress. *Br J Rheumatol* 1998; **37**: 870–3.

9 Hannan MT, Anderson JJ, Pincus T, Felson DT. Educational attainment and osteoarthritis: differential associations with radiographic changes and symptom reporting. *J Clin Epidemiol* 1992; **45**: 139–47.

10 Hurley MV, Scott DL, Rees J, Newham DJ. Sensorimotor changes and functional performance in patients with knee osteoarthritis. *Ann Rheum Dis* 1997; **56**: 641–8.

11 Messier SP, Royer TD, Craven TE, *et al.* Long-term exercise and its effects on balance in older, osteoarthritic adults: results from the fitness, arthritis and seniors trial (FAST). *JAGS* 2000; **48**: 131–8.

12 Sharma L, Pai Y. Impaired proprioception and osteoarthritis. *Current Opinion in Rheumatology* 1997; **9**: 253–8.

13 Van Baar ME, Assendelft WJJ, Dekker J, *et al.* Effectiveness of exercise in patients with osteoarthritis of the hip or knee. A systematic review of randomised clinical trials. *Arthritis Rheum* 1999; **42**: 1361–9.

14 Ettinger WH Jr, Burns R, Messier SP, *et al.* A randomized trial comparing aerobic exercise and resistance exercise with a health education program in older adults with knee osteoarthritis. *JAMA* 1997; **277**: 25–31.

15 Van Baar ME, Dekker J, Oostendorp RAB, *et al.* The effectiveness of exercise therapy in patients with osteoarthritis of the hip or knee. A randomised clinical trial. *J Rheumatol* 1998; **25**: 2432–9.

16 Börjesson M, Robertson E, Weidenheilm L, *et al.* Physiotherapy in knee osteoarthritis: effect of pain on walking. *Physiotherapy Res In* 1996; **1**: 89–97.

17 Kovar PA, Allegrante JP, MacKenzie CR, *et al.* Supervised fitness walking in patients with osteoarthritis of the knee. A randomised controlled trial. *Annals of Internal Medicine* 1992; **116(7)**: 529–34.

18 O'Reilly SC, Muir KR, Doherty M. Effectiveness of home exercise on pain and disability from osteoarthritis of the knee: a randomised controlled trial. *Ann Rheum Dis* 1999; **58**: 15–19.

19 O'Reilly SC, Ratcliffe K, Lones AC, *et al.* A simple exercise programme can improve pain in knee osteoarthritis: a community based randomised controlled trial. *Arthritis Rheum* 1999; **42**(Suppl): S404.

20 Prochaska J, DiClemente C, Norcross J. In search of how people change: applications to addictive behaviors. *Am Psychol* 1992; **47**: 1102–14.

21 Oakley A, France-Dawson H, Fullarton D, *et al.* Preventing falls and subsequent injury in older people. *Effective Health Care* 2000, **2**: 1–16.

22 Felson DT. Weight and osteoarthritis. *J Rheumatol* 1995; **22**: 7–9.

3 | The health benefits of physical activity for patients with chronic heart failure

Andrew Clark

Introduction

Chronic heart failure is a quiet epidemic. Little is heard about it as compared with, for example, cancer. Yet it affects approximately one percent of the population, and carries with it a poor prognosis; the five year survival in men is only 25%. It affects predominantly older people and seriously reduces quality of life.[1] The dominant symptom is exercise intolerance usually due to fatigue, breathlessness, or both. The efficacy of pharmacological treatments to relieve symptoms and improve outcome is well established. The study of non-pharmacological treatment has had less active support, particularly from the drug industry. Nevertheless, exercise training is gradually gaining acceptance as a useful part of the general management of heart failure.

Background and safety

There is much in common between heart failure and detraining (see Table 1). Much of the evidence suggests that secondary, peripheral changes rather than the primary, central haemodynamic changes of the

Table 1. Comparison of heart failure physiology with the 'detrained' state.

Variable	Detraining	Heart failure
Heart rate	↑	↑
Heart rate variability	↓	↓
Muscle wasting	↑	↑
Sympathetic activation	↑	↑
Renin-angiotensin activation	↑	↑
Loss of oxidative enzymes	↑	↑
Exercise capacity	↓	↓

diseased heart, are responsible for the generation and progression of symptoms of heart failure.[2] Exercise training has been shown to be of benefit in patients with ischaemic heart disease. It thus seemed reasonable to try the effects of training for patients with chronic heart failure. Traditional advice to patients with chronic heart failure had been to avoid physical exertion[3] despite the fact that few studies had specifically addressed rest as a therapy. Those studies that had were conducted in the 1960s before modern therapies were available. There was a high drop out rate from these early studies, and a high mortality.[4,5] Would exercise training be less hazardous?

Some early anxieties were raised by Jugdutt's influential study, testing the effects of training early after an anterior myocardial infarction.[6] This study reported an increase in left ventricular dysfunction and a worsening of symptoms (despite an increase in exercise capacity) after training. However, these findings have not been replicated. A larger study (the EAMI study) showed no difference in left ventricular function between a trained group and controls following myocardial infarction.[7] Training has been found to be safe in patients with ischaemic heart disease, some of whom are highly likely to have had left ventricular dysfunction.[8,9] So far in training studies in heart failure, there have been no reports of serious adverse events.

Controlled trials

In the early, uncontrolled studies, training appeared beneficial. The first controlled studies were reported in 1988.[10] Two studies using a crossover design produced more convincing evidence that training improves the exercise capacity of patients with chronic heart failure.[11,12] Nevertheless, it is important to bear in mind that fewer than 1000 patients have been trained in randomised controlled studies. These patients have all been highly selected. They are younger than most patients with chronic heart failure, and tend to be highly motivated to follow their exercise prescription. Bearing in mind these caveats about the generalisability of the findings, it is important to consider some of the trials in more detail.

One of the first trials to excite interest in training in heart failure was that of Coats et al from Oxford.[11,13] It was a crossover study, in random order, comparing training using cycle exercise for 20 minutes, five days a week for eight weeks against restricted activity in 17 men with moderate to severe stable chronic heart failure. The investigators reported an 18% increase in exercise capacity, a reduction in ventilatory response to exercise and an improvement in the sympathetic-vagal imbalance in heart failure, with an increase in heart rate variability and reduction in noradrenaline spillover.

A second randomised crossover study in 18 patients with severe heart failure produced similar results.[12] The training consisted of supervised treadmill and cycle training together with general exercises. There was an improvement in exercise capacity, reduction in ventilatory response to exercise and improvements in symptom scores after only three weeks of training.

Other authors have demonstrated similar results with improvements in exercise capacity of the order of 20%.[14] From the patients' perspective, training improves their quality of life[15] and increases exercise tolerance. The latter is accompanied by an increase in exercise efficiency – that is a reduction in the energy cost of walking.[16] Other benefits are summarised in Table 2. It is interesting to note that benefits are seen in many of the variables that are associated with a poor prognosis. The effect of training on prognosis is unknown, but trials are in progress to investigate this.

Table 2. Effects of exercise training in patients with chronic heart failure.

Variable		Variable	
Quality of life	↑	Metabolism	
		Cytochrome C positive	
Exercise		mitochondria	↑
Peak exercise capacity	↑	Phosphocreatine depletion	↓
Submaximal endurance	↑	Phosphocreatine resynthesis	↑
Anaerobic threshold	↑	Citrate synthase	↑
Ventilatory response	↓		
		Autonomic	
Skeletal muscle		Sympathetic	↓
Bulk	↑	Vagal	↑
Strength	↑	Heart rate variability	↑
Endurance	↑		
Ergoreflex	↓		
		Prognosis	**?**

How does training improve exercise capacity in heart failure?

Cardiac output and muscle blood flow

The effects of training on central haemodynamic function are not certain. The majority of training studies have not reported any great change in cardiac function, although there is usually a reduction in heart rate at submaximal work loads. Cardiac output at maximal exercise tends to increase, and some have interpreted this phenomenon as the mechanism by which training works. This suggestion, however, is probably incorrect.

If a patient performs maximal treadmill exercise, and then at peak exercise is asked to perform additional arm exercise, cardiac output increases further. This suggests that it is not cardiac output that limits exercise capacity in heart failure.

Furthermore, the post-training association between an increased maximal cardiac output and an increased maximal work rate need not be causal. In a progressive exercise test, cardiac output at peak exercise will increase after training, simply because exercise can be continued for longer and therefore to a greater intensity.

It may be that training 're-educates' the vasculature generally so that a limited blood flow is better distributed to exercising muscle. In rat experiments, training (swimming) improved flow-mediated dilation of peripheral arteries.[17] In human heart failure, training improves endothelial function and endothelium dependent vasodilation.[18]

Skeletal muscle and the 'ergoreflex'

As exercise proceeds, the working muscle signals to the brain, and generates a ventilatory response. In patients with heart failure, this 'ergoreflex' is much greater than normal. Careful observation suggests that the enhanced ergoreflex may also explain the increased sympathetic nervous system activity of heart failure.

It is not known why this reflex is enhanced. There may be a link with other changes in muscle. Loss of skeletal muscle bulk occurs early in the course of the disease. Muscle metabolism is abnormal with early onset of acidosis during exercise, and slower re-synthesis of adenosine triphosphate at the end of exercise. Muscle is functionally abnormal with reduced strength and endurance.

Training at least partially reverses these abnormalities with improvements in muscle function and metabolism (see Table 2). The effects on the ergoreflex are particularly interesting. Piepoli *et al* were the first to demonstrate the ergoreflex was enhanced in heart failure[19] and that the ergoreflex activity relates strongly to exercise capacity and the ventilatory response to exercise.[20] Training results in decreased ergoreflex activity.[19] This observation suggests a mechanism by which training works (Fig 1). Improving peripheral, rather than central, factors, may be the important step.

Training regimen

The appropriate training regimen for heart failure is not yet clear. As noted above, the studies have used carefully selected, motivated patients

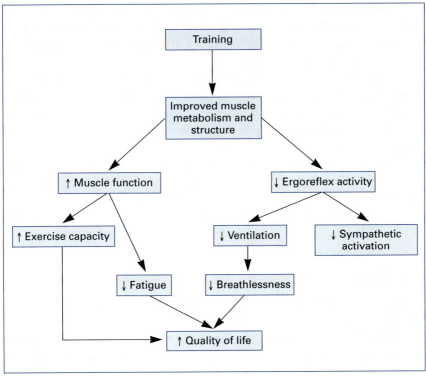

Fig 1. Possible route by which training may benefit patients with heart failure. An important role is allotted to improvements in the periphery rather than to any benefits in haemodynamics.

with stable disease, little in the way of comorbidity and younger than most patients with heart failure. Exercise training programmes have been closely supervised.

Intensity

Training has usually been performed at 60–80% of maximal exercise capacity. In practice, this is an uncomfortable intensity of exercise. There have been some studies demonstrating benefits at ≤50% of maximum. Indeed, some benefit can be demonstrated using just local muscle group training.

Frequency

The available evidence suggests that training must be for at least 20 minutes, at least three times a week.

Type of exercise

Endurance aerobic training, such as cycling, walking or running and rowing have principally been used. A resistive component to the training regimen results in greater increases in muscle bulk, although how this translates to symptomatic benefit is unclear.

Duration

Training benefits develop over approximately 16 weeks, reaching a plateau. Thereafter, if training stops, there is a rapid return to the pre-training state. If training is maintained, then so are the benefits, at least up to one year.[21] It is likely that training will have to be continued indefinitely.

Supervision

In academic studies, training tends to have been closely supervised. Even where there has been training at home, patients have returned at regular intervals for 'top-up' sessions under supervision. Exercise training does appear to be safe, so that there may be no medical need to supervise closely. Nevertheless, the benefits of training are related to compliance[13] and this may be better with some supervision.

Logistics

On present knowledge, unstable patients should not train, particularly those with active disease such as myocarditis or acute intercurrent illness, and those with peripheral oedema. Any patient with symptoms suggestive of ischaemia at low workload should be considered for revascularisation prior to training. An initial (supervised) exercise test is important to help determine baseline exercise capacity and to demonstrate safety in terms of ischaemia and exercise induced arrhythmia or hypotension. Training should then start gradually, and build up.

Herein lies a large problem. When a new drug is introduced that demonstrates symptomatic or survival benefit for patients with heart failure, it is relatively straightforward for the doctor to prescribe it, and for the patient to take it. Prescribing exercise is more difficult as it demands far more from the patients. In addition, there are difficulties for health services in the fact that heart failure is so common that it will be practically impossible to offer supervised training for all. For some patients, particularly the more frail, initial supervision is essential. This allows patients to discover the sort of exercise they can do, and to build some confidence in themselves.

For other patients, the physician can offer more general advice. Exercise should be encouraged. Brisk walking or cycling are appropriate, at a level where the patient is aware of becoming somewhat breathless, for about 20 minutes, at least three times a week.

Conclusions

For patients with chronic heart failure, exercise training offers improvements in quality of life and exercise capacity over and above those offered by optimal drug intervention. It improves many of the pathophysiological features associated with an adverse prognosis. The effects of training on mortality are not yet known. Far from limiting patients' activity, the evidence suggests that we should strongly encourage patients to exercise regularly.

References

1 Stewart AL, Greenfield S, Hays RD, *et al.* Functional status and well-being of patients with chronic conditions. *JAMA* 1989; **262**: 907–13.

2 Clark AL, Poole-Wilson PA, Coats AJS. Exercise limitation in chronic heart failure: The central role of the periphery. *J Am Coll Cardiol* 1996; **28**: 1092–102.

3 Braunwald E (ed). *Heart disease (3e).* Philadelphia: WB Saunders Co, 1988.

4 Burch GE, Walsh JJ, Black WC. Value of prolonged bed rest in management of cardiomegaly. *JAMA* 1963; **183**: 81–7.

5 Burch GE, McDonald CD. Prolonged bed rest in the treatment of ischemic cardiomyopathy. *Chest* 1971; **60**: 424–30.

6 Jugdutt BI, Michorowski BL, Kappagoda CT. Exercise training after anterior Q wave myocardial infarction: Importance of left ventricular function and topography. *J Am Coll Cardiol* 1988; **12**: 362–72.

7 Gianuzzi P, Tavazzi L, Temporelli PL, *et al,* for the EAMI Study group. Long-term physical training and left ventricular remodelling after anterior myocardial infarction (EAMI) trial. *J Am Coll Cardiol* 1993; **22**: 1821–9.

8 Oldridge NB, Guyatt GH, Fisher ME, Rimm AA. Cardiac rehabilitation after myocardial infarction: Combined experience of randomized clinical trials. *JAMA* 1988; **260**: 945–50.

9 O'Connor GT, Buring JE, Yusuf S, *et al.* An overview of randomized trials of rehabilitation with exercise after myocardial infarction. *Circulation* 1989; **80**: 234–44.

10 Sullivan MJ, Higginbotham MB, Cobb FR. Exercise training in patients with severe left ventricular dysfunction: hemodynamic and metabolic effects. *Circulation* 1988; **78**: 506–16.

11 Coats AJS, Adamopoulos S, Meyer T, *et al.* Physical training in chronic heart failure. *Lancet* 1990; **335**: 63–6.

12 Meyer K, Schwaibold M, Westbrook S, *et al.* Effect of short-term exercise training and activity restriction on functional capacity in patients with severe chronic congestive heart failure. *Am J Cardiol* 1996; **78**: 1017–22.

13 Coats AJS, Adamopoulos S, Radaelli A, *et al.* Controlled trial of physical training in chronic heart failure: exercise performance, hemodynamics, ventilation and autonomic function. *Circulation* 1992; **85**: 2119–31.

14 Sullivan MJ, Higgenbotham MB, Cobb FR. Exercise training in patients with severe left ventricular dysfunction: hemodynamic and metabolic effects. *Circulation* 1988; **78**: 506–16.

15 Belardinelli R, Georgiou D, Cianci G, Purcaro A. Randomized, controlled trial of long-term moderate exercise training in chronic heart failure: Effects on functional capacity, quality of life, and clinical outcome. *Circulation* 1999; **99**: 1173–82.

16 Beneke R, Meyer K. Walking performance and economy in chronic heart failure patients pre and post exercise training. *Eur J Appl Physiol* 1997; **75**: 246–51.

17 Varin R, Mulder P, Richard V, *et al.* Exercise improves flow mediated vasodilatation of skeletal muscle arteries in rats with chronic heart failure. *Circulation* 1999; **99**: 2951–7.

18 Hambrecht R, Fiehn E, Weigl C, *et al.* Regular physical exercise corrects endothelial dysfunction and improves exercise capacity in patients with chronic heart failure. *Circulation* 1998; **98**: 2709–15.

19 Piepoli M, Clark AL, Volterrani M, *et al.* Contribution of muscle afferents to the hemodynamic, autonomic, and ventilatory responses to exercise in patients with chronic heart failure: effects of physical training. *Circulation* 1996; **93**: 940–52.

20 Piepoli M, Ponikowski P, Clark AL, *et al.* A neural link to explain the 'muscle hypothesis' of exercise intolerance in chronic heart failure. *Am Heart J* 1999; **137**: 1050–6.

21 Kavanagh T, Myers MG, Baigrie RS, *et al.* Quality of life and cardiorespiratory function in chronic heart failure: effects of 12 months' aerobic training. *Heart* 1996; **76**: 42–9.

4 | The health benefits of physical activity for patients with obesity and diabetes

Patrick Sharp

Introduction

As society becomes increasingly sedentary with the development of labour saving devices, there is growing concern that fitness levels in the general population are falling. Presumably as a consequence of this, obesity is an increasing problem. In the US, a series of large scale surveys has been carried out between the years 1971–1991.[1] These have demonstrated that in the years 1971–1975, the prevalence of obesity was 25%, whereas in 1988–1991 this rose to 33.3%. In certain ethnic groups, this figure was considerably higher. A similar trend has been noted in the UK between 1980 and 1993, although the prevalence of obesity was less than in the US,[2] with 13% of males and 16% of females having a body mass index (BMI) greater than 30 kg/m^2 (Fig 1).

The health hazards of obesity have been reviewed,[4] demonstrating an increase in plasma lipids and blood pressure with increasing BMI, the

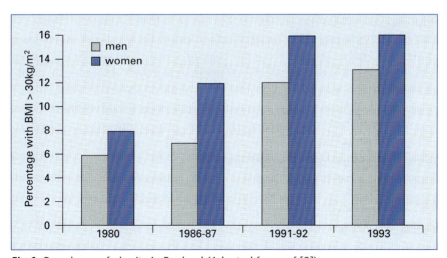

Fig 1. Prevalence of obesity in England (Adapted from ref [3]).

25

steeper part of the curve being above a level of approximately $30kg/m^2$. Type 2 diabetes is strongly associated with obesity, an association being found with the degree of obesity, with the duration of obesity and with central distribution of body fat. In the Health Professional Study,[5] there was a low risk of diabetes in men with a BMI below $24kg/m^2$, rising exponentially such that a BMI of $35kg/m^2$ was associated with a 40-fold relative risk. A similar relationship was found in women in the Nurses Health Trial,[6] with the lowest risk at a BMI of below 22 kg/m^2, rising 60-fold with a BMI above $35kg/m^2$.

Hyperinsulinaemia is closely associated with obesity. The sequence of events has been well characterised. With the development of obesity, there is an associated decrease in glucose removal, and the development of insulin resistance has been demonstrated with glucose clamp studies. Insulin resistance is associated with an increase in very low-density lipoprotein (VLDL) triglyceride synthesis, a decrease in glucose transporters in muscle and with lower glucokinase levels in muscle. These effects may be mediated by reduced insulin effectiveness in promoting activity of these two components of glucose metabolism, and also reduced activity of peroxisome proliferating activator receptor-γ, an area of current interest as the site of newer therapeutic modalities. Eventually, as pancreatic insulin activity is no longer able to maintain elevated insulin levels, overt diabetes becomes apparent.

Physical activity in the prevention of diabetes

Physical activity is an attractive possibility for ameliorating the effects of obesity on glucose metabolism. The effect of physical activity on improvement in insulin sensitivity has been well documented, although there is still considerable debate whether improved insulin sensitivity is a short lived effect relating to the last bout of activity, and whether it simply relates to weight loss associated with habitual activity.[7,8] However, it seems likely that the insulin sensitizing effect of physical activity is independent of weight loss since studies have shown that even if body weight is not normalised, exercise can bring about improvements in glucose tolerance.[9,10] In clinical practice, there is a well recognised progression of impaired glucose tolerance to diabetes,[11] with 3.2% of patients with impaired fasting glucose and 5.4% with impaired glucose tolerance progressing over a three year study period (relative risks of 5.6 and 9.6 respectively). Studies of the effect of exercise on the progression of impaired glucose tolerance to overt diabetes have shown very significant benefits but have emphasised the need for the increase in activity to be continued.[12–14]

Physical activity and vascular risk in diabetes

The huge increase in vascular disease associated with type 2 diabetes was recently highlighted by the UK Prospective Diabetes Study.[15,16] Control of blood glucose and of blood pressure brought about improvements in vascular risk, but even in the intensively treated groups, the risk was still much greater than in the non-diabetic population. There is, therefore, great potential for exercise as an additional risk modifier in patients with diabetes. However, the majority of patients with type 2 diabetes are very sedentary in their habits. In a recent study, 54.6% of participants with diabetes reported zero minutes of physical activity in an average week,[17] despite recommendations that exercise must be a 'high priority' for individuals with diabetes.[18]

Patients with type 2 diabetes demonstrate both peripheral and hepatic insulin resistance. During exercise, peripheral glucose uptake increases more than hepatic glucose production, resulting in a net fall in blood glucose.[19] At the same time, plasma insulin levels fall, suggesting improved insulin sensitivity, and these changes may persist for 12–16 hours after the exercise session.[20,21] In practical terms, a fall in HbA1 of 1.0–1.5% after six weeks training has been reported.[22] As in the non-diabetic population, exercise has a beneficial effect on the lipid profile and other markers of vascular risk.[23,24]

A recent study has provided evidence in terms of hard end-points for the benefits of exercise in type 2 diabetes.[25] In a group of 1,263 men with type 2 diabetes, followed for an average of 12 years, fitness was graded by both self-reported assessment and measured by a maximal exercise test. The relative risk of death in the unfit was approximately twice that of the fitter group (Fig 2).

How much exercise?

As in the non-diabetic population, recent interest has focused on the level of exercise required to bring about improved physical and metabolic fitness in subjects with diabetes. In a study of subjects with type 2 diabetes, a 12-week walking programme was found to bring about significant benefits.[26] Likewise, both aerobic exercise and resistance exercise have been shown to be beneficial, fuelling the argument that it may be weight loss which is the important factor.[27] On the basis of these and other studies, the recommendation is that exercise of moderate intensity should be undertaken on most days for 30 minutes.[18] It may also be more encouraging to refer to 'physical activity' rather than 'exercise', since the latter term may be a disincentive to many!

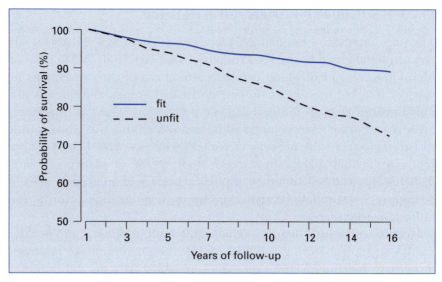

Fig 2. Mortality curves in men with type 2 diabetes, graded as either fit or unfit.[25]

Special considerations for patients with type 1 diabetes

For patients with insulin treated diabetes, exercise-related improvement in glycaemic control is more difficult to attain. This arises from the complicated problems of achieving optimal blood glucose and blood insulin levels at the onset of exercise. Too much insulin, and hypoglycaemia will ensue: insufficient, and hepatic glucose output will rise beyond the scope of increased peripheral utilisation. Nonetheless, there have been many reports of patients with insulin dependent diabetes undertaking strenuous exercise without problem,[28,29] and it should be the aim of those caring for subjects with diabetes to encourage them to overcome the practical difficulties associated with exercise and insulin therapy. Care should be taken to counsel patients on the dangers of hypoglycaemia which can occur many hours after cessation of exercise as a result of reduced glycogen stores. Despite the difficulty in improving blood glucose control in insulin dependent diabetes, improvements in the lipid profile with exercise are apparent.[30]

Conclusion

All published data point towards a beneficial effect of moderate exercise, not only in healthy individuals, but also in those at increased vascular risk, such as those with obesity and diabetes. Areas of debate continue, such as the relative contributions of physical activity itself and of the associated weight loss. Irrespective of the mechanism, however, the evidence of benefit is overwhelming. Perhaps research should now focus on practical means of encouraging and enabling physical activity by patients with obesity and diabetes.

References

1   Kuczmarski RJ, Flegal KM, Campbell SM, *et al.* Increasing prevalence of overweight among US adults: The National Health and Nutrition Examination Surveys, 1960 to 1991. *JAMA* 1994; **272**: 205.

2   VanItallie TB. Prevalence of obesity. *Endocrinol Metab Clin North America* 1996; **25**(4): 887–905.

3   Nutrition and Obesity Task Forces. Obesity: Reversing the increasing problem of obesity in England. London: Department of Health,1995.

4   Bray GA. Health hazards of obesity. *Endocrinol Metab Clin North America* 1996; **25**(4): 907–19.

5   Chan JM, Rimm EB, Colditz GA, *et al.* Obesity, fat distribution and weight gain as risk factors for clinical diabetes in men. *Diabetes Care* 1994; **17**: 961–9.

6   Colditz GA, Willett WC, Rotnitzky A, *et al.* Weight gain as a risk factor for clinical diabetes mellitus in women. *Ann Intern Med* 1995; **122**: 481–6.

7   Gulve E, Cartee G, Zierath J, *et al.* Reversal of enhanced muscle glucose transport after exercise. Roles of insulin and glucose. *Am J Physiol* 1990; **259**: E685.

8   Rice B, Janssen I, Hudson R, Ross R. Effects of aerobic or resistance exercise and/or diet on glucose tolerance and plasma insulin levels in obese men. *Diabetes Care* 1999; **22**: 684–91.

9   Krotkiewski M, Bylund-Fallenius A, Holm J, *et al.* Relationship between muscle morphology and metabolism in obese women. The effects of long term physical training. *Eur J Clin Invest* 1983; **5**: 5.

10 Tremblay A, Despres J, Maheux J, *et al.* Normalisation of the metabolic profile in obese women by exercise and a low fat diet. *Med Sci Sports Exerc* 1991; **23**: 1326.

11 Charles MA, Fontbonne A, Thibult N, *et al.* Risk factors for NIDDM in white population. *Diabetes* 1991; **40**: 796–9.

12 Eriksson KF, Lindgarde F. Prevention of type 2 (non-insulin dependent) diabetes by diet and physical exercise. The 6 year Malmo feasibility study. *Diabetologia* 1991; **34**: 891–8.

13 Pan X-r, Li G-w, Hu Y-H, *et al.* Effects of diet and exercise in preventing NIDDM in people with impaired glucose tolerance. *Diabetes Care* 1997; **20**: 537–44.

14 Wing RR, Venditti E, Jakicic JM, *et al.* Lifestyle intervention in overweight individuals with a family history of diabetes. *Diabetes Care* 1996; **21**: 350–9.

15 UK Prospective Study Group. Intensive blood-glucose control with sulphonylureas or insulin compared with conventional treatment and risk of complications in patients with type 2 diabetes (UKPDS 33). *Lancet* 1998; **352**: 837–53.

16 UK Prospective Study Group. Tight blood pressure control and risk of macrovascular and microvascular complications in type 2 diabetes: UKPDS 38. *Br Med J* 1998; **317**: 703–13.

17 Hays LM, Clark DO. Correlates of physical activity in a sample of older adults with type 2 diabetes. *Diabetes Care* 1999; **22**: 706–12.

18 American Diabetes Association. Diabetes mellitus and exercise. *Diabetes Care* 1997: **20**: 1908–12.

19 Minuk HL, Vranic M, Marliss E, *et al.* Glucoregulatory and metabolic response to exercise in obese non-insulin dependent diabetes. *Am J Physiol* 1981; **240**: E458–64.

20 Koivisto VA, DeFronzo RA. Exercise in the treatment of type II diabetes. *Acta Endocrinol* 1984; **262**(suppl): 107–11.

21 Devlin JT, Hirshman M, Horton ED, Horton ES. Enhanced peripheral and splanchnic insulin sensitivity in NIDDM men after single bout of exercise. *Diabetes* 1987; **36**: 434–9.

22 Schneider SH, Amorosa LF, Khachadurian AK, Ruderman NB. Studies on the mechanism of improved glucose control during regular exercise in type 2 (non-insulin dependent) diabetes. *Diabetologia* 1984; **26**: 355–60.

23 Ruderman NB, Ganda OP, Johansen K. The effect of physical training on glucose tolerance and plasma lipids in maturity-onset diabetes. *Diabetes* 1979; **28**(suppl 1): 89–92.

24 Skarfors ET, Wegener TA, Lithell H, Selinus I. Physical training as treatment for type II (non-insulin dependent) diabetes in elderly men. A feasibility study over 2 years. *Diabetologia* 1987: **30**: 930–3.

25 Wei M, Gibbons LW, Kampert JB, Nichaman MZ, Blair SN. Low cardiorespiratory fitness and physical inactivity as predictors of mortality in men with type 2 diabetes. *Ann Intern Med* 2000; **132**: 605–611.

26 Walker KZ, Piers LS, Putt RS, *et al.* Effects of regular walking on cardio-vascular risk factors and body composition in normoglycaemic women and women with type 2 diabetes. *Diabetes Care* 1999; **22**: 555–61.

27 Rice B, Janssen I, Hudson R, Ross R. Effects of aerobic or resistance exercise and/or diet on glucose tolerance and plasma insulin levels in obese men. *Diabetes Care* 1999; **22**: 684–91.

28 Meinders AE, Willekins FLA, Heere LP. Metabolic and hormonal changes in IDDM during long distance run. *Diabetes Care* 1988; **11**: 1–7.

29 Sane T, Helve E, Pelkonen R, Koivisto VA. The adjustment of diet and insulin dose during long term endurance exercise in type I (insulin dependent) diabetic men. *Diabetologia* 1988; **31**: 35–40.

30 Wallberg-Henriksson H, Gunnarsson R, Henriksson , *et al.* Increased peripheral insulin sensitivity and muscle mitochondrial enzymes but unchanged blood glucose control in type 1 diabetics after physical training. *Diabetes* 1982; **31**: 1044–50.

5 | The health benefits of physical activity for a healthier old age

Archie Young

Introduction

The health benefits of habitual physical activity are considerable,[1,2] and are at least as great in later life (Fig 1).[3] This review is intended both to guide the reader to the extensive evidence that supports this statement and to highlight areas ripe for further investigation.

> *'Exercise of some kind or other is almost essential to the preservation of health in persons of all ages – but in none more so than in the old.'*

Fig 1. The opinion of Dr. Daniel MacLachlan, physician and surgeon to the Royal Hospital, Chelsea, 1840–1863, and author of *A practical treatise on the diseases and infirmities of advanced life.*[4]

Health is a 'state of complete physical, mental and social well-being'.[5] A healthier old age, therefore, requires less risk of disease, better physical and mental function, richer opportunities for social interaction and a greater sense of control and responsibility for one's own health and well-being (Fig 2). Participation in physical activity contributes to all five of these inter-related determinants of health.

Absence of disease

The most prominent disease-prevention benefits of habitual physical activity concern common conditions of particular importance in later life (eg ischaemic heart disease, stroke, hypertension, maturity onset diabetes, and osteoporosis).[1,2] It is clear that most of these disease prevention benefits still operate for those who are physically active in later life.[6–11] This is despite the theoretical possibility that selective premature mortality of those sedentary people who are genetically most vulnerable to the hazards of inactivity might have reduced the impact of the protective effect of later life activity.

31

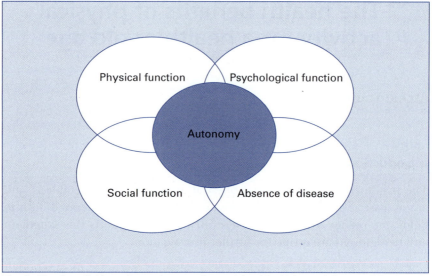

Fig 2. The interlinking determinants of good health (Adapted from ref [63] with permission).

An area which remains uncertain is the effect on mortality (especially cardiovascular and cerebrovascular) of the new adoption of physical activity in later life. Existing longitudinal studies have limited statistical power to answer this question because of the small numbers of old people surviving in the study and making such a transition. Harvard alumni changing from <1500kcal/week to ≥1500kcal/week of walking, stair climbing and sports or recreational activities between 1962/66 and 1977, showed a 28% reduction in all-cause mortality between 1977 and 1988.[12] The published analysis includes consideration of the men grouped according to their ages in 1977. The benefit of changing to a more active lifestyle appears to apply across the full age range (but the confidence limits are not provided for individual age bands). The men in the oldest group (aged 75–84 in 1977) were aged between 60–83 when they changed their lifestyle. They then averaged an additional 9 months of life between 1977 and 1988 (or age 90), compared with those who remained sedentary.

The Copenhagen male study, however, has raised the possibility that men changing from a sedentary to a physically more active lifestyle when aged 64–74, might experience twice as many ischaemic heart disease events as those who remain sedentary.[13] This apparent increase in relative risk was not statistically significant but, until better evidence is available, it cannot be ignored. Perhaps the only way to settle this issue will be by pooling data from several large, long-term longitudinal epidemiological studies.

Physical function

Counteracting the effects of ageing

At advanced ages, the greatest importance of physical activity to health shifts from the prevention of disease to the preservation of physical performance in activities of everyday life (Fig 3). The special importance of habitual physical activity at advanced ages is its ability to preserve functional independence by counteracting some of the age-related decline in physical performance. The muscle cachexia (sarcopenia) of ageing brings weakness and fatiguability, even in the absence of disease. The age-associated differences seen in healthy elderly men and women imply deterioration of static strength at 1–2% per year,[14] of explosive power (as exerted in a single fast movement against a resistance) at 3–4% per year,[14] and of aerobic power (ie maximal oxygen consumption) at some 1% per year.[15] These losses put elderly people (especially women, with their lower power/weight ratios) dangerously close to functionally important thresholds, needing only a small further impairment to lose the ability to perform some everyday task, or to render it so fatiguing as to be unpleasant to perform.[16]

For example, if the ratio of the explosive power of the extensors of the dominant lower limb to body weight is less than 1.5W/kg, some people will not be able to mount a 30cm step (without a hand rail) and fewer than 30% will be able to manage a 50cm step.[17] In the English National Fitness Survey, almost half (47%) of community-dwelling women aged 70–74 (but only 14% of the men of the same age) had an explosive power/weight ratio below the 1.5W/kg threshold (Fig 4).[18] Men averaged a 20 year advantage over the women in their values for this functionally important characteristic.

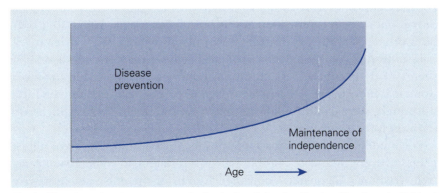

Fig 3. The changing importance of physical activity for the health of an individual (Reproduced from ref [18] with permission).

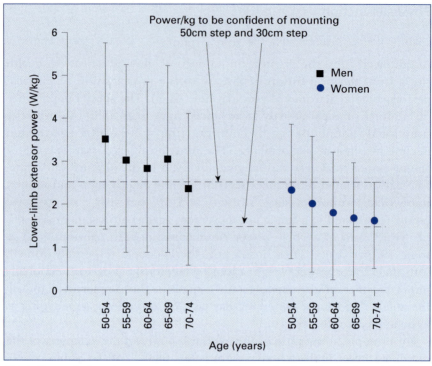

Fig 4. Lower limb extensor power (better limb, standardised for body weight) in a representative sample of men and women aged 50–74 (mean ±2SD). (Data from the English National Fitness Survey. Reproduced from ref [18] with permission).

Comfort during sustained walking requires that the oxygen cost is less than 50% of the individual's maximal oxygen uptake. The oxygen cost of walking at 3mph on the level is 12.5 ml/kg/min. Thus, to be comfortable during a sustained walk at 3mph requires that one has a maximal oxygen consumption of at least 25 ml/kg/min.[18] In the English National Fitness Survey, more than three-quarters (80%) of women aged 70–74 (but only 35% of men) fell below this functional threshold (Fig 5).[18] Women fell below this threshold value at least 15 years earlier than men. By age 80, it seems likely that even just 2mph (in comfort) is impossible for most women.[15] Indeed, even just sitting still all day is probably as fatiguing for a detrained 80-year-old female patient as an eight hour shift in heavy industry is for a young man.[15]

Fortunately, octogenarians undergoing physical training, experience gains in strength and in aerobic power equivalent to some 10–20 years 'rejuvenation'. Adequately controlled studies of the effects of resistance training on strength have confirmed that this is true for healthy octogenarians,[19] for residents in institutional care,[20,21] and for those who

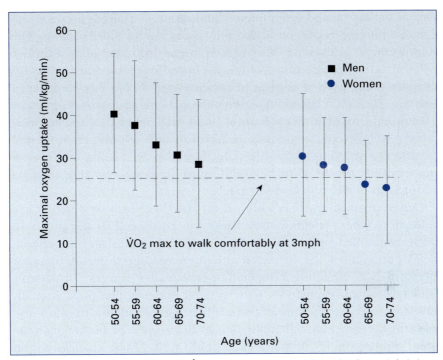

Fig 5. Maximal oxygen uptake ($\dot{V}O_2$max) (standardised for body weight) in a representative sample of men and women aged 50–74 (mean ±2SD). (Data from the English National Fitness Survey. Reproduced from ref [18] with permission).

have previously sustained a hip fracture.[22] For improvements in aerobic power produced by endurance training, it applies to healthy octogenarians[23] and septuagenarians.[24,25]

Only a few studies have attempted directly to compare young and old adults' responses to the same relative intensity of training stimulus. Young and old subjects appear to have broadly similar percentage responses for strength,[26] for muscle size,[27] and for maximal (or peak) oxygen uptake.[28–30] As a result, the absolute intensity of exercise required to improve an older person's physical performance may be so low that it includes many everyday activities. Not only does this reduce costs, it also makes it easier to ensure that the functional benefits, which may be highly specific to the actions performed in training,[19,31] are relevant to everyday life.[31]

Counteracting the effects of disease

This refers to the amelioration of the functional impact of established, disease-related impairments in patients with angina, heart failure, chronic airflow limitation, and intermittent claudication.[1,2] There is no reason to suppose that this reduction in disability is any less for older patients. The improvements in exercise capacity seen in patients undergoing a cardiac rehabilitation programme which included exercise training were, proportionally, at least as great in patients aged 75+ as in patients aged less than 60 years.[32] (In addition, the older patients also showed similar or greater improvements in cholesterol (total, HDL and LDL), triglycerides, anxiety, depression, somatisation, hostility, and self-perceived mental health, energy, general health, pain, function, well-being and overall quality of life.) It would be helpful if future studies also analyse the data for patients of different ages separately.

Other promising areas which merit further study and which are relevant to older patients include Parkinson's disease (PD) and stroke. In an uncontrolled study of patients with PD, an intensive, but general, activity programme was associated with numerous improvements in motor performance, including PD-specific performance scores.[33] In patients with established hemiparesis, there is good evidence that physiologically effective exercise training is feasible[34] and that walking training also reduces the excessive metabolic demands imposed by the hemiparetic gait.[35] Future studies should seek to confirm that these changes are, in fact, associated with the expected functional benefit.[36]

Falls

Falls are common in old age and are associated with considerable physical, psychological and social morbidity. Systematic reviews are divided in their opinion on the effectiveness of exercise as an intervention.[37,38] Some of the positive evidence suggests quite dramatic potential for benefit.[39] Other reports, however, claim positive findings on rather thin evidence. For example, the meta-analysis of the FICSIT ('Frailty and Injuries: Cooperative Studies of Intervention Techniques') studies was interpreted by the authors as indicating a beneficial effect of exercise in the prevention of falls.[40] This seems an over optimistic reading of the findings as the various control groups differed from the corresponding exercise groups in ways other than just participation in an exercise programme. There is, therefore, no certainty that exercise was an important factor in the multifactorial interventions. On the other hand, the FICSIT evidence does look encouraging for the prevention of falls by the frequent practice of activities which make demands on balance.[40]

If, as seems likely, there are circumstances in which some forms of physical activity are beneficial in preventing falls, why has this not been a consistent finding in all studies? Confounding results may have arisen as a result of too little attention being given to the specificity of training. For example, balance training improves balance (but not strength) and strength training improves strength (but not balance).[41] Or perhaps the exercise intervention in some studies provided practice in movements which failed adequately to reproduce the real life, fall-inducing situation. It is striking that, in one of the FICSIT studies, it was Tai Chi, rather than computerised balance training, which reduced falls and fear of falling.[42] Another important possibility is that newly adopted physical activity by someone with a history of falls may have the potential to result in more falls[43] (perhaps especially if frail exercisers are given insufficient initial guidance).

Psychological function

Cognition

Life-long habitual physical activity can be assumed to provide substantial, indirect protection against cognitive decline through its known beneficial effects against atherosclerotic arteriopathy, hypertension and diabetes. This presumably explains the cognitive advantage of active subjects which is apparent in cross-sectional comparisons.[44,45] Nevertheless, there is only limited, longitudinal evidence that physical training in old age reverses, or offers protection against, cognitive decline.[44-47]

It seems likely that the performance of a bout of activity has a short-term arousal effect, potentially improving performance in some tests of cognitive function.[48] It will be important to ensure that future longitudinal studies of the effects of physical training in old age have a design that adequately excludes this effect. It is not clear whether this was the case in the two studies which appear to show cognitive benefit from an increase in habitual activity sustained for 6 or 12 months.[46,47]

Depression

There is ample anecdote and face validity (and varying degrees of evidence) that a bout of physical activity may enhance mood. Many studies have attempted to test the longer term effect of physical activity on the mood of older people but such studies are difficult to design and to interpret.[49] Nevertheless, two small studies do suggest a therapeutically useful effect of physical activity in the treatment of depression.[50,51] In a rather larger study, the effects of aerobic exercise were compared with those of antidepressive medication (sertraline) in the treatment of patients (aged 50–77 years) meeting DSM IV criteria for major depressive disorder.[52] Over 16 weeks of treatment, the two treatments were associated with equal improvements in depression scores. Unfortunately, however, there was no placebo control or attention control group. These will be essential features of future studies; the ethical difficulties should not be insurmountable.

Other factors contributing to psychological well-being

Some other problems, in areas where physical function and psychological function overlap, may all be ameliorated by an increased level of habitual activity. These include back pain (in osteopenic women aged 50–70),[53] knee pain (in people, of mean age 69 years, limited by osteoarthritis),[54] poor sleep (in people, mean age 61, with moderate sleep complaints),[55] and sleep disturbance in depression (in people of mean age 71).[51] These changes would be valuable at any age but could be crucial for the quality of later life.

Social function

It seems likely that many of the improvements in mood and in self-perceived well-being reported anecdotally may owe more to group socialisation than to physical activity *per se*. This interpretation receives some support from studies in which the exercise group and the control group were given a similar degree of attention and social contact and showed similar gains. This emphasises the importance of organising group exercise sessions in such a way that ample opportunities are provided for socialisation.[56] It would be short-sighted to neglect the importance of the potential opportunities provided by exercise classes for socialisation (including socially acceptable physical contact) and for the renewal of a contracting social network. There is even epidemiological evidence consistent with the possibility that maintaining a rich social network reduces the risk of cognitive decline.[57,58]

Autonomy

Increased participation in physical activity is one of the most important public health goals in the developed world. For the individual, however, it offers much more than this; it offers a way of taking control and directly influencing personal health and well-being. The well-being of older people is enhanced by measures which increase their sense of control, especially in circumstances (such as major health challenges or institutional care) which might otherwise foster a sense of helplessness.[59,60] There is also anecdotal support for the view that participation in physical activity can be a valuable means of expressing autonomy while regaining and reinforcing the sense of control.[61] Indeed, the role of physical activity for a healthier old age may even extend to a greater use of rehabilitation exercise in palliative care.[62] Anecdote and discussion suggest that the potential benefits are considerable; there is a great need for formal evaluation of this unexplored area.

Acknowledgments

I am grateful to Mrs Carol Talbot for bibliographic assistance and to Drs Gillian Mead and Carolyn Greig for helpful criticism.

References

1   Bouchard C, Shephard RJ, Stephens T (eds). *Physical Activity, Fitness, and Health: International Proceedings and Consensus Statement.* Champaign: Human Kinetics, 1994.

2   US Department of Health and Human Services. *Physical Activity and Health: A Report of the Surgeon General.* Atlanta, GA: US Department of Health and Human Services, Centers for Disease Control and Prevention, National Center for Chronic Disease Prevention and Health Promotion, 1996.

3   Cavanagh P, Evans WJ, Fiatarone M, *et al.* Exercise and physical activity for older adults. *Med Sci Sports Exerc* 2000; **30**: 992–1008.

4   MacLachlan D. *A Practical Treatise on the Diseases and Infirmities of Advanced Life.* London: John Churchill & Sons,1863.

5   World Health Organization. *Constitution of the World Health Organization: Annexe 1. The First Ten Years of the World Health Organization.* Geneva: WHO, 1958.

6   Hakim AA, Curb D, Petrovitch H, *et al.* Effects of walking on coronary heart disease in elderly men. The Honolulu Heart Programme. *Circulation* 1999; **100**: 9–13.

7   Wannamethee SG, Shaper AG. Physical activity and the prevention of stroke. *J Cardiovasc Risk* 1999; **6**: 213–6.

8   Sacco RL, Gan R, Boden-Albala B, *et al.* Leisure-time physical activity and ischemic stroke risk: the Northern Manhattan Stroke Study. *Stroke* 1998; **29**: 380–7.

9   Burchfiel CM, Sharp DS, Curb JD, *et al.* Physical activity and incidence of diabetes: the Honolulu Heart Program. *Am J Epidemiol* 1995; **141**: 360–8.

10 Cononie CC, Graves FE, Pollock ML, *et al.* Effect of exercise training on blood pressure in 70- to 79-yr-old men and women. *Med Sci Sports Exerc* 1991; **23**: 505–11.

11 Feskens EJ, Loeber JG, Kromhout D. Diet and physical activity as determinants of hyperinsulinemia: the Zutphen Elderly Study. *Am J Epidemiol* 1994; **140**: 350–60.

12 Paffenbarger RS, Kampert JB, Lee I-M, *et al.* Changes in physical activity and other lifeway patterns influencing longevity. *Med Sci Sports Exerc* 1994; **26**: 857–65.

13   Hein HO, Suadicani P, Sørensen H, Gyntelberg F. Changes in physical activity level and risk of ischaemic heart disease. *Scand J Med Sci Sports* 1994; **4**: 57–64.

14   Skelton DA, Greig CA, Davies JM, Young A. Strength, power and related functional ability of healthy people aged 65-89 years. *Age Ageing* 1994; **23**: 371–7.

15   Malbut-Shennan KM, Greig C, Young A. Aerobic exercise. In: Evans JG, Williams TF, Beattie BL, *et al* (eds). *Oxford Textbook of Geriatric Medicine.* Oxford: Oxford University Press, 2000.

16   Young A. Exercise physiology in geriatric practice. *Acta Med Scand* 1986; **(Suppl)711**: 227–32.

17   Levy DI, Young A, Skelton DA, Yeo A-L. Strength, power and functional ability. In: Passeri M (ed). *Geriatrics '94.* Rome: CIC Edizioni Internazionali, 1994.

18   Skelton D, Young A, Walker A, Hoinville E. *Physical Activity in Later Life; a Further Analysis of the Allied Dunbar National Fitness Survey and the Health Education Authority National Survey of Activity and Health.* London: HEA, 1999.

19   Skelton DA, Young A, Greig CA, Malbut KE. Effects of resistance training on strength, power, and selected functional abilities of women aged 75 and older. *J Am Geriatr Soc* 1995; **43**: 1081–7.

20   Fiatarone MA, O'Neill EF, Ryan ND, *et al.* Exercise training and nutritional supplementation for physical frailty in very elderly people. *N Engl J Med* 1994; **330**: 1769–75.

21   McMurdo MET, Rennie LM. Improvements in quadriceps strength with regular seated exercise in the institutionalised elderly. *Arch Phys Med Rehabil* 1994; **75**: 600–3.

22   Sherrington C, Lord SR. Home exercise to improve strength and walking velocity after hip fracture: a randomized controlled trial. *Arch Phys Med Rehabil* 1999; **78**: 208–12.

23   Malbut-Shennan KE, Dinan SM, Young A. Aerobic training can increase maximal oxygen uptake in women over 80. *Med Sci Sports Exerc* 1998; **30**: S138.

24   Warren BJ, Nieman DC, Dotson RG, *et al.* Cardiorespiratory responses to exercise training in septuagenarian women. *Int J Sports Med* 1993; **14**: 60–5.

25   Hagberg JM, Graves JE, Limacher M, *et al.* Cardiovascular responses of 70–79 year old men and women to exercise training. *J Appl Physiol* 1989; **66**: 2589–94.

26   Welle S, Thornton C, Statt M. Myofibrillar protein synthesis in young and old human subjects after three months of resistance training. *Am J Physiol* 1995; **268**: E422–7.

27   Welle S, Totterman S, Thornton C. Effect of age on muscle hypertrophy induced by resistance training. *J Gerontol* 1996; **51A**: M270–5.

28   Makrides L, Heigenhauser GJ, Jones NL. High-intensity endurance training in 20- to 30- and 60- to 70-yr-old healthy men. *J Appl Physiol* 1990; **69**: 1792–8.

29   Stratton JR, Levy WC, Cerqueira MD, *et al.* Cardiovascular responses to exercise. Effects of aging and exercise training in healthy men. *Circulation* 1994; **89**: 1648–55.

30   Malbut-Shennan KE, Dinan SM, Verhaar H, Young A. *Personal Communication.*

31   Skelton DA, McLaughlin AW. Training functional ability in old age. *Physiotherapy* 1996; **82**: 159–67.

32   Lavie CJ, Milani RV. Effects of cardiac rehabilitation and exercise training programs in patients ≥75 years of age. *Am J Cardiol* 1996; **78**: 675–7.

33   Reuter I, Engelhardt M, Stecker K, Baas H. Therapeutic value of exercise training in Parkinson's disease. *Med Sci Sports Exerc* 1999; **31**: 1544–9.

34   Potempa K, Lopez M, Braun LT, *et al.* Physiological outcomes of aerobic exercise training in hemiparetic stroke patients. *Stroke* 1995; **26**: 101–5.

35   Macko RF, DeSouza CA, Tretter LD, *et al.* Treadmill aerobic exercise training reduces the energy expenditure and cardiovascular demands of hemiparetic gait in chronic stroke patients. *Stroke* 1997; **28**: 326–30.

36   Duncan P, Richards L, Wallace D, *et al.* A randomized, controlled pilot study of a home-based exercise program for individuals with mild and moderate stroke. *Stroke* 1998; **29**: 2055–60.

37   Oakley A, France-Dawson M, Fullerton D, *et al.* Preventing falls and subsequent injury in older people. *Effective Health Care* 2000; **2(4)**: 1–16.

38   Gillespie LD, Gillespie WJ, Cumming R, *et al.* Interventions for preventing falls in the elderly. *The Cochrane Database of Systematic Reviews* 2000; **1**: 1–49.

39   Campbell AJ, Robertson MC, Gardner MM, *et al.* Randomised controlled trial of a general practice, home based exercise programme for falls prevention in elderly women. *Br Med J* 1997; **315**: 1065–9.

40   Province MA, Hadley EC, Hornbrook MC, *et al.* The effects of exercise on falls in elderly patients. *J Amer Med Ass.* 1995; **273**: 1341–7.

41   Wolfson L, Whipple R, Derby C, *et al.* Balance and strength training in older adults: intervention gains and tai chi maintenance. *J Am Geriatr Soc* 1996; **44**: 498–506.

42   Wolf SL, Barnhart HX, Kutner NG, *et al.* Reducing frailty and falls in older persons: an investigation of tai chi and computerized balance training. *J Am Geriatr Soc* 1996; **44**: 489–97.

43   Ebrahim S, Thompson PW, Baskaran V, Evans K. Randomized placebo-controlled trial of brisk walking in the prevention of postmenopausal osteoporosis. *Age Ageing* 1997; **26**: 253–60.

44   Dustman RE, Emmerson R, Shearer D. Physical activity, age and cognitive-neuropsychological function. *J Aging Phys Act* 1994; **2**: 143–81.

45   Chodzko-Zajko W, Moore KA. Physical fitness and cognitive functioning in aging. *Exerc Sport Sci Rev* 1994; **22**: 195–220.

46   Williams P, Lord SR. Effects of group exercise on cognitive functioning and mood in older women. *Aust NZ J Public Health* 1997; **21**: 45–52.

47   Kramer AF, Hahn S, Cohen NJ, *et al.* Ageing, fitness and neurocognitive function. *Nature* 1999; **400**: 418–9.

48   Netz Y, Jacob T. Exercise and the psychological state of institutionalized elderly. *Perceptual Motor Skills* 1994; **79**: 1107–18.

49   O'Connor PJ, Aenchbacher III LE, Dishman RK. Physical activity and depression in the elderly. *J Aging Phys Act* 1993; **1**: 34–58.

50   McNeil JK, LeBlanc EM, Joyner M. The effect of exercise on depressive symptoms in the moderately depressed elderly. *Psychol Aging* 1991; **6**: 487–8.

51   Singh NA, Clements KM, Fiatarone MA. A randomized controlled trial of the effect of exercise on sleep. *Sleep* 1997; **20**: 95–101.

52   Blumenthal JA, Babyak MA, Moore KA, *et al.* Effects of exercise training on older patients with major depression. *Arch Intern Med* 1999; **159**: 2349–56.

53   Bravo G, Gauthier P, Roy P-M, *et al.* Impact of a 12-month exercise program on the physical and psychological health of osteopenic women. *J Am Geriatr Soc* 1996; **44**: 756–62.

54 Ettinger WH, Burns R, Messier SP, *et al.* A randomized trial comparing aerobic exercise and resistance exercise with a health education program in older adults with knee osteoarthritis. *J Amer Med Ass* 1997; **277**: 25–31.

55 King AC, Oman RF, Brassington GS, *et al.* Moderate-intensity exercise and self-rated quality of sleep in older adults. *J Amer Med Ass* 1997; **277**: 32–7.

56 Young A, Dinan S. Active in later life. In: McLatchie G, Harries M, Williams C, King J (eds). *ABC of Sports Medicine.* London: BMJ Publishing 2000.

57 Berkman LF. Which influences cognitive function: living alone or being alone? *Lancet* 2000; **355**: 1291–2.

58 Fratiglioni L, Wang H-X, Ericsson K, *et al.* Influence of social network on occurrence of dementia: a community-based longitudinal study. *Lancet* 2000; **355**: 1315–9.

59 Rodin J. Aging and health: effects of the sense of control. *Science* 1986; **233**: 1271–6.

60 Wolinsky FD, Stump TE. Age and the sense of control among older adults. *J Gerontol* 1996; **51B**: S217–20.

61 Cohn AH. Chemotherapy from an insider's perspective. *Lancet* 1982; **1**: 1006–9.

62 Tookman A. *Personal Communication.*

63 Kennie DC, Dinan S, Young A. Health promotion and physical activity. In: Tallis R, Fillit H, Brocklehurst JC (eds). *Geriatric Medicine and Gerontology.* New York: Churchill Livingstone, 1998.

6 | Delivering an exercise prescription for patients in primary care

Steve Iliffe, Sharon See Tai, Mairi Gould and Paul Smith

Introduction

Promoting physical activity is becoming a mainstream concern in general practice, with growing numbers of 'exercise prescription' schemes[1,2] and increasing interest amongst practitioners in methods of encouraging patients to change their behaviour. Efforts in general practice settings to promote exercise as a public health solution for future ill-health, such as an inoculation against heart disease, have been disappointing, and there is an argument that investment in exercise promotion in primary care is a waste of resources. However, exercise as a form of therapy for particular problems may be more effective, and more popular with professionals and patients alike. There is a danger that the uncertainties about the effectiveness of exercise promotion may inhibit practitioner involvement in research and development into encouraging more physical activity, just at a time when it is needed.

This chapter will review the important issues around prescribing or referring for exercise therapy in primary care. We will discuss which patient groups are likely to benefit most, which individuals are most likely to take up and sustain programmes of physical activity, and how the potential risks of physical activity can be minimised. Findings from a study of patients taking up exercise referrals will be used to illustrate these points.

The referral process will be outlined, for referral must be appropriate and the exercise therapist must be an expert, and should be provided with a comprehensive account of the reasons for the referral, and who should feed back findings and outcomes to the primary care practitioner.

Will exercise prescription in general practice make any difference to health and to the use of health services in the long-term? We will not know for sure until results of trials and case-control studies are available, but there is a research agenda with which practitioners can engage in the course of developing exercise promotion, and this will be considered.

Prescribing exercise

The scale of physical inactivity in the UK is so great that no specialist service could hope to make an impact upon it. Only half of all adults are physically active at least three times a week, and fewer than this exercise to recommended levels to maintain cardiovascular fitness.[3] The consequence is low levels of fitness in the population. About 40% of older adults (65–74 years) engage in so little physical activity that their health is jeopardised and their quality of life reduced.[3] Walking is less common as a mode of transport, especially for children, and walked journeys are shorter.[4] Since physical inactivity contributes to heart disease risk to the same extent as smoking, we may face a major public health problem as an increasingly inactive population ages. The social norm in an increasingly automated society is to remain sedentary, whereas smoking is increasingly expensive, increasingly difficult in many public places and widely regarded as both unhealthy and unpleasant. Increasing physical activity is in this sense counter-cultural, and poses a significant challenge to those trying to put public health principles into practice.

Physical activity behaviour is determined by combinations of social, environmental and personal variables that prevent any single method of promoting change from being effective in practice populations. Nevertheless, there are some characteristics of people and of processes that appear to influence the uptake of advice about physical activity. The individual's readiness to change[5] is important, and only those seriously intent on increasing their physical activity will seek a method that is acceptable, accessible, appropriate, effective and affordable. Premature advice on the need for increased activity in those committed to inaction may promote resistance and defensiveness, and instructions about action are likely to be premature for many patients still contemplating or preparing for a change in their behaviour.[6] Stimuli to action may be important (the poster in the waiting room may matter more than we think, for some individuals) and reinforcement of behaviour through positive gain (increased physical well-being, success in completion of programmes, a sense of mastery) or avoidance of distress (reduction in anxiety or depression symptoms) appears to improve adherence to activity programmes. Self-monitoring of activity (in the form of a diary) allows the individual to establish a personal package of stimuli and reinforcements, and in one study increased the frequency of physical activity.[7] Social support, including that provided by health professionals, may also function as a package of stimuli and reinforcements, and has been found to be associated with sustained change in activity levels over a two year period.[8] Self-efficacy, the individual's perception of their own capability, predicts physical activity level[9] and is determined by previous experience, vicarious experience, encouragement by others and the interpretation of physiological responses to exercise as positively healthy or hazardous.[10]

This assessment appears complex, and perhaps impossible to fit into the short consultations of general practice, but this impression may be false. Contact with patients over a period of time may be helpful in gaining an understanding of individuals' readiness to change, self-efficacy and support, as well as environmental issues like safety and sites for activity. One question for primary care practitioners is how do we collect and collate this information?

Does the ability of general practitioners, and other members of primary care teams, to accumulate knowledge about patients put them in a good position to change their activity behaviour? The evidence is not encouraging. In one study general practitioners and practice nurses rank physical inactivity as less significant than smoking, hypertension and a high fat diet in contributing to heart disease risk, and had a sketchy knowledge of the impact of exercise on other medical conditions.[11] Enrolment of patients in physical activity programmes tends to be slow[12] and draws on no more than one percent of the potential population.[13] The only primary care based trial to show significant increases in the levels of physical activity did not directly involve primary care staff in the intervention.[14] Although community based exercise programmes appear to be effective in increasing activity in US populations,[15] an approach to a population through general practice in the UK has not shown such effects.[16] Prescribing exercise, in the sense of providing detailed recommendations to individuals or of helping them to make use of local leisure facilities, may seem a logical approach to the public health problem of inactivity, but we have little evidence that it produces sustained changes in behaviour. This does not imply that exercise prescription is not worthwhile, only that its commissioning could not be supported by current evidence. The evidence is enough to justify further exploration of different approaches, and also to warrant investigation of exercise programmes as specific forms of therapy for common clinical problems.

Exercise uptake and adherence

Many individuals appear to warrant intervention against a risk factor for disease, or as treatment for an existing condition, but not all will accept the intervention or use that treatment regularly, systematically or even at all. Rational prescribing of or referral for exercise depends not only on correct identification of the need and potential for exercise, but also on correct understanding of the individual's commitment to pursue an exercise programme. How can the practitioner know which individuals will take up and continue physical activity until it is effective? We used a pilot exercise prescription project in inner London to identify the characteristics of individuals who adhered to a complete exercise programme.

Patients in fourteen inner city practices had access to programmes of moderate intensity aerobic exercise at local leisure centres, provided that they fell into a low risk category but were deconditioned, overweight, smokers, stressed, depressed, or at risk from heart disease because of family history or raised cholesterol, or having diet-controlled diabetes, mild to moderate osteoarthritis, or osteoporosis. A standardised referral form, including information about the aims of referral to the programme was used for all referrals, and was presented by patients at their initial consultation with a fitness consultant. A supervised, tailored exercise programme of twenty one-hour sessions was organised for each patient referred. A fuller description of the programme[17], with the views of the health professionals involved[18], has been reported elsewhere.

Anonymous referral and demographic data, and BMI, were collected from successive patients who attended the initial fitness consultation at the leisure centres over a period of 18 months. The referral form contained a section for referrers' aims, which were agreed between the professional making the referral and the patient. Two members of the research group independently categorised the recorded aims before agreeing on final categories, and patient attendance at the exercise programme was analysed using these categories. The final six categories used for this analysis were: weight reduction and lifestyle change; improving fitness; reducing stress, anxiety and depression; relieving physical and musculo-skeletal problems; gaining psychosocial benefits (such as improving self esteem); and reducing heart disease risk factors.

During the 18 months of the study 152 people started the exercise programme, of whom 71% were women and 29% were men. The age range for women was 16–75 years and for men 19–74 years, but 66% of women and 71% of men were under the age of 50 years. Weight loss was the most common referral aim (13 men and 41 women), and reduction in heart disease risk factors the least common (seven men and five women)

Only 16% of women and 21% of men completed the programme. There were no significant differences between adherers and drop-outs in sex or BMI, but adherers were significantly older. The mean age of adherers was 50 years compared with 44 years for drop-outs ($p=0.026$).

Completion of the programme was associated with the referral aims of 'reducing heart disease risk factors' in women and 'reducing stress, anxiety and depression' in both sexes.

The finding that older people have higher adherence rates is consistent with other studies[19] and supports the practice of targeting older rather than younger patients for exercise referral. In recent exercise prescription schemes the tendency has been to refer younger women for weight control (exactly the groups who failed to complete the programme in our study).

Case management and exercise promotion

Once the demographic and psychological characteristics of those most likely to take up and continue with increased physical activity are known, practitioners have to make a decision how to intervene with their patients. We now know that direct instruction in the benefits of exercise has no impact on behaviour but that linking physical activity as a form of primary or secondary prevention to the management of existing health problems in multi-dimensional interventions may be fruitful. There is no evidence that use of specialist exercise therapists in primary care settings increases uptake of or adherence to physical activity. The tasks of identifying suitable patients and prescribing exercise or referring for exercise therapy therefore lie with the practitioner, who needs to build them into brief consultations about current or anticipated health problems. Decisions have to be taken about whether primary prevention is needed (exercise prescription) or secondary intervention (referral for exercise therapy). How can this be done in a limited time?

The answer probably includes the following basic principles:

1. Knowledge about the individual's health, understanding of exercise benefits and motivation needs to be built up. This needs to be done over a period of time, making recording the impressions of the practitioner important. The importance of the social dimension of exercise needs to be known for each individual.

2. The recommended daily dose of moderate physical activity should be described as 30 minutes of effort sufficient to make the individual slightly warm and slightly breathless. Strength, suppleness and better balance need different approaches, which are the province of the exercise specialist.

3. This activity should be built into daily routines wherever possible, not added on, unless it is a form of therapy for a specific problem.

4. A mixture of different physical activities tailored to individuals is the best option.

5. Safety probably matters more for exercise as therapy than it does for exercise prescription. It entails alerting the therapist to any hazards in the medical history or medication, warning of any conditions or treatments that could influence activity, and where necessary, educating the patient in warning signs. The difficulty for the practitioner is that the benefits of increased physical activity are likely to be greatest amongst those with some existing medical problem, like angina, diabetes, arthritis or high blood pressure.

How can practitioners apply these principles, either to exercise prescription or to referral for exercise therapies? Once patients ready to change are identified (principle 1, above) an approach like that shown in Box 1 appears to have the greatest chance of promoting change in activity behaviour. Many of these nine points correspond to the principles listed above.

Box 1
Nine components of a programme for promoting physical activity (Adapted from ref [20]).

- ▶ Written description of benefits of exercise
- ▶ Elicit expectations of exercise
- ▶ Make expectations realistic
- ▶ Assessment of self-efficacy
- ▶ Instruction on safe exercising
- ▶ Identify enjoyable settings
- ▶ Self-monitoring (heart rate monitoring, diaries)
- ▶ Reinforcement – telephone contact, later consultations
- ▶ Plan for interruptions to exercise programme

This list is too extensive to work through in any but the exceptional consultation in primary care, but this does not preclude its insertion in the written medical record or appearance as a template on the computer record. The necessary elements of an exercise prescription would therefore be written material on exercise, advice tailored to individuals and a mechanism for reinforcing the advice.

Physical activity can be a useful therapy for chronic backpain[21] and in established heart disease,[22] but requires specialist assessment and treatment design. Referral for exercise therapy requires a referral process of the kind described by Dinan and Young,[23] in principle no different from referral to any other specialist service. This should include the aim of referral, major medical problems, medication, precautions to be taken, specific activities that should be considered, and some sense of what the individual's motivation is like. In addition, it asks specifically about potential problems such as those listed in Box 2.

Just like any other specialist, those providing exercise programmes as therapy should let the referring practitioner know the outcomes of their interventions.

Box 2
Potential problems in providing exercise as therapy (Adapted from ref [23]).

▶ Heart rate not being an indicator of exercise intensity
▶ Impairment of balance
▶ Impairment of alertness and cognition
▶ Urinary frequency
▶ Suppression of pain
▶ Susceptibility to:
  – asthma
  – angina
  – arrhythmias
  – hypotension
  – hypoglycaemia
  – infection
  – joint pain
  – osteoporosis
  – abnormal muscle tone

A research and development agenda

Promotion of physical activity in primary care is not an easy subject, for there are many thick guidelines supported by thin evidence. Targeting older age groups and those most likely to benefit because of existing medical problems looks more hopeful as a strategy than population wide attempts at primary prevention of heart disease. Working out who will take up advice on physical activity seems to be complicated, and requires accumulated knowledge of individuals, systematically collected and carefully appraised. Designing exercise programmes requires specialist assessment of individuals, except perhaps for the kind of primary prevention approach that seems to work in the US but not yet in UK.

Large scale trials to test more intense interventions to promote activity, particularly among older people in the community, will no doubt happen. Practitioners keen to develop exercise promotion but not involved in such trials may find that smaller scale studies of interventions targeted at common but important conditions are a feasible way of exploring this potentially powerful alternative therapy.

References

1 Chapman T. *Directory of GP-referred Exercise Schemes in England.* Chicester: School of Health Studies, Chichester Institute of Higher Education, 1996.

2 Riddoch C, Puig-Ribera, Cooper A. *Effectiveness of Physical Activity Promotion Schemes in Primary Care: A Review.* London: Health Education Authority, 1998.

3 Health Education Authority and Sports Council. *Allied Dunbar National Fitness Survey 1992.* London: HEA, 1992.

4 Department of the Environment. *Focus on Personal Travel.* London: HMSO, 1998.

5 Prochaska JO, DiClemente CC, Norcross JC. In search of how people change: applications to addictive behaviours. *Am Psychol* 1992; **47**: 1102–11.

6 Rollnick S, Heather N, Bell A. Negotiating behaviour change in medical settings: the development of brief motivational interviewing. *J Mental Health* 1992; **1**: 25–37.

7 King A , Barr Taylor C, Haskell WL, DeBusk RF. Strategies for increasing early adherence to and long term maintainance of home based exercise training in healthy middle aged men and women. *Am J Cardiol* 1988; **61**: 628–32.

8 Sallis JF, Melbourne F, Hovell C, *et al.* Explanation of vigorous physical activity during two years using social learning variables *Soc Sci Med* 1992; **34**: 25–32.

9 Garcia AW, King AC. Predicting long term adherence to aerobic exercise: a comparison of two models. *J Sport Exercise Psychol* 1991; **13**: 394–410.

10 Clark NM, Becker MH. Theoretical models and strategies for improving adherence and disease management. In: Sumaker SA, Schron EB, Ockene JK, McBee WL (eds). *The Handbook of Health Behaviour Change.* New York: Springer, 1998.

11 Gould MM, Thorogood M, Iliffe S, Morris JN. Promoting physical activity in primary care: measuring the knowledge gap. *Health Educ J* 1995; **54**: 304–11.

12 Hillsdon M. Promoting physical activity: issues in primary care. *Int J Obesity* 1998; **22**: S52–4.

13 Fox K, Biddle S, Edmunds L, *et al.* Physical activity promotion through primary health care in England. *Br J Gen Pract* 1997; **47**: 367–9.

14 Stevens W, Hillsdon M, Thorogood M, McArdle D. Cost-effectiveness of a primary care based physical activity intervention in 45–74 year old men and women: a randomised controlled trial. *Br J Sports Med* 1998; **32**: 236–41.

15 Hillsdon M, Thorogood M, Antiss T, Morris J. Randomised controlled trials of physical activity promotion in free living populations: a review. *J Epidemiol Community Health* 1995; **49**: 448–53.

16 Harland J, White M, Drinkwater C, *et al.* The Newcastle exercise project: a randomised controlled trial of methods to promote physical activity in primary care. *Br Med J* 1999; **319**: 828–32.

17 See Tai S, Gould M, Smith P, Iliffe S. Promoting physical activity in general practice: should prescribed exercise be free? *J R Soc Med* 1999; **92**: 65–7.

18 Smith P, Gould MM, See Tai S, Iliffe S. Exercise as therapy? Results from group interviews of practices involved in an inner-London prescription for exercise scheme. *Health Educ J* 1996; **55**: 439–46.

19 Stockport Health Commission. *Exercise on Prescription – Does it Work? A Detailed Evaluation Report of the Pilot Scheme in Stockport.* Stockport Health Commission,1993.

20 Barr Taylor C, Miller NH. *Principles of Behaviour Change. American College of Sports Medicine's Resource Manual for Exercise Testing and Prescription.* Baltimore: Williams & Wilkins, 1998.

21 Baker P. Group support is crucial to success. *Br Med J* 2000; **320**: 1472.

22 McMurdo M. Excluded patients should be encouraged to take up exercise. *Br Med J* 2000; **320**: 1473.

23 Young A, Dinan S. Active in later life. In: *ABC of Sports Medicine (2e).* London: BMJ Publications, 2000.

7 | Delivering an exercise prescription for vulnerable older patients

Susie Dinan

Introduction

Vulnerable elderly patients are a frail but heterogeneous group. In addition to hospital in-patients, they include most of those who reside in nursing homes, retirement and residential homes but also some of those who live at home. Many are over 80 years of age, and most are seated for most of the day. Although some still mobilise independently indoors (perhaps with a frame), many need assistance from another person when walking outdoors or, indeed, just to get around indoors. Many have multiple pathologies and medications, considerable limitation in functional mobility and in the ability to carry out activities of everyday living. Breathlessness, arthritis, contractures and postural instability are common. At least 20% have cognitive impairment.

Even very vulnerable older patients can exercise safely, provided that the exercise programme is appropriately designed and adapted to their needs. This chapter reviews the adaptations that must be made to exercise practice to ensure optimal benefits with minimal risk for vulnerable, older patients. The chapter will also look at the role of the doctor in facilitating an individually tailored exercise programme for these patients.

Substantial health benefits are available to most older individuals. They include the prevention of disease, the preservation of everyday functional abilities and the facilitation of psychosocial benefits. For those who are severely disabled, movement (even in the absence of a training effect) still contributes to the prevention of the medical complications of immobility. This chapter does not discuss the evidence for these benefits (which is covered elsewhere[1]), concentrating instead on how both the content and the delivery of the exercise must be adapted in order to ensure that it is safe and effective for even the most vulnerable older patient.

Guidelines for the programming of exercise for the healthy older person wishing to engage in regular moderate to vigorous physical activity have already been published.[2] What is missing from these guidelines are specific recommendations for meeting the needs of the frailer, older patient, viz:

i   pre-exercise assessment procedures, including the role of the referring clinician,

ii types and progressions of exercise for vulnerable older patients with different chronic and degenerative diseases,

iii the specialist knowledge and competencies required by those supervising activity for these vulnerable individuals.

However, an increasing number of respected authorities are addressing these issues.[3-7] The recommendations that follow are a combination of specific research outcomes, published guidelines for programming exercise (for healthy, older participants), and recommendations which have evolved in the course of interdisciplinary collaborations with both fitness professionals and health professionals who have considerable experience and expertise in various aspects of working with frail and vulnerable older patients.

The role of the doctor

Healthy older people who plan just to increase their daily walking or other light or moderate intensity activities may need no special evaluation and are recommended simply to discuss their plans with their general practitioner. On the other hand, referral to an exercise professional is appropriate if the person is likely to need help with motivation, supervision, monitoring, choice of duration, frequency, time and type of physical activity directed at specific health and functional outcomes.[8] The frailest and most vulnerable elderly patients routinely require referral to specialist exercise professionals. Their individually tailored exercise programmes should be based on an 'enabling', pre-exercise, medical review, ie one that emphasises benefits rather than risks and facilitates safer, more effective participation.[3,4,9]

The referring doctor's contribution is highly important and includes four key responsibilities:[3,8]

1. To identify the pathologies that are present and ensure that they, and all medications, are accurately communicated to the exercise practitioner.

2. To highlight any ways these may influence the safety or comfort of physical activity (for example susceptibility to angina, shortness of breath, arrhythmias, joint pain, confusion or any medication-induced effects such as suppression of pain, production of a bradycardia unrepresentative of exercise effort, increased susceptibility to postural hypotension etc.) Any specifically contraindicated exercises and activities and any information the patient has been given should also be included.

3. To educate the exercise participant in the early recognition of symptoms that might indicate the exercise programme was, in some way unsuitable for them and their chronic pathologies. For example the patient with osteoarthritic knees should be taught to recognise and respect an increase in pain, stiffness or swelling. The trained exercise practitioner will continue this educational process in relation to specific exercises and day-to-day fluctuations in health and function.

4. To monitor and review the patient's progress, encouraging feedback from patients and a productive dialogue with the exercise practitioner.

Clinical responsibility therefore, rests with the referrer. The responsibility for applying the clinical information to the administration, design, delivery and ongoing evaluation of the patient's exercise programme, on the other hand, rests with the exercise instructor or exercise practitioner service.

The role of the exercise practitioner – pre-exercise assessment

Because of the prevalence of chronic and degenerative disease, assessment before participation is essential when working with vulnerable, older patients. It is important to emphasise, however, that the aim of assessment is not to exclude those at risk but rather to ensure the inclusion of each individual in an appropriate exercise programme (Box 1).

Effective pre-exercise assessment should include appraisal of the individual's:

- health history (including current medications)
- functional abilities (by history and by direct observation)
- activity history
- current interests
- preferences
- means
- readiness to exercise.

The health history should be obtained from the referring physician or clinician, with the patient's written consent. It is important to identify all pathologies, medications and physical limitations and to establish the ways in which these affect the performance of everyday actions and, if known, exercise.[3]

The exercise practitioner personally should then take the individual's health history and compare it with the information received from the referrer. The health history should include the location, nature and

---

Box 1
Pre-exercise assessment
(Adapted from ref [16])

Pre-exercise assessment ensures that even patients with:
- complex, multiple disabilities
- cardiac and circulatory disease
- respiratory disease
- joint problems and diseases
- osteoporosis
- postural instability
- impairment in cognition
- depression, or anxiety, or social isolation
    will benefit from suitably adapted exercise programmes.

However,

The absolute contraindications to exercise in vulnerable older patients are:
- Uncontrolled angina
- Uncontrolled resting SBP>180 mmHg or resting DBP>100 mmHg
- Significant drop in BP during exercise
- Uncontrolled resting tachycardia >100 bpm
- Unstable or acute heart failure
- Uncontrolled acute systemic illness (eg pneumonia)
- Uncontrolled visual or vestibular disturbances
- Recent injurious fall without a medical examination
- People with proven inability to comply with the recommended adaptations to the exercise programme

---

precipitants of any pain, dizziness, breathlessness or fatigue, and a list of all medications. The clinical exercise practitioner is trained to recognise which medications might have effects that are relevant to the safe, comfortable conduct of exercise.

The level of functional mobility is a key factor in developing an individually tailored exercise programme for an older patient. Functional reach, timed 'up and go', flexibility, tandem gait and other validated measures[10] should be recorded, along with observations of pain, breathlessness and instability during the functional tests. The exercise practitioner will also make their own measurements of lying and standing blood pressure. Only occasionally is there a role for exercise stress testing, eg in order to determine physiological safety thresholds. This would depend on the level and type of activity intended, the patient's medical details, and the availability of appropriately trained personnel.[11]

The role of the exercise practitioner – safe and effective programming for older people

'Programming physical activity for older people requires more care and more expertise than for any other age group with only a fine line separating effective from dangerous procedures'.[12]

Best practice with the most vulnerable begins with the conscientious observance of the guidelines for designing and delivering exercise programmes for any older participant. Further adaptations must then be applied to session aims, content, programming and teaching techniques to ensure optimal benefit for each individual patient.

Session structure

For all older participants sessions should start and finish gradually.

Warm-up

A longer, gradual warm-up (15 minutes) is suggested, to ensure adequate cardiovascular and articular adaptation. A sound warm-up comprises:

i   moves that use the large muscle groups of the arms and, wherever possible, the legs in a continuous, rhythmical way, gradually increasing the size, range and pace of movements;

ii specific joint mobility exercises performed from a stable base;

iii controlled stretching activities.

Chair and/or standing alternatives should be used as appropriate. Additional time should be added if the temperature is colder than usual.

Warm-down

A longer, gradual warm-down (10 minutes) is also suggested for older participants, to preserve central venous return and allow muscle and skin vasodilatation to return to resting levels.[3] This takes account of the increased risk of postural hypotension and related falls in this patient group. Continuous, rhythmic exercises similar to those used in the warm-up give way to the practice of more specific, controlled activities such as stretching, balance training, floorwork and relaxation, depending on the needs of the group.

Further adaptations for vulnerable older patients

Frail patients may not be able to exercise continuously for as long as 20 minutes, but multiple shorter bouts of exercise may be possible. The efficacy of this approach has not been formally established in elderly people but there is evidence that two to three bouts of 10–15 minutes of moderate aerobic exercise produces rather similar effects to one single, longer bout in healthy, younger people.[13,14] In our dementia care programme, three short bouts of daily exercise (2 short walks and a ball game, that all begin gently, then build up and finally wind down gradually) are better tolerated than a single, longer session. In our primary care sessions the level of frailty is such that the journey to the practice is often a workout in itself. A 15-minute rest is therefore scheduled before and after the session to allow for recovery. Meeting and chatting before the session, and close observation of participants during a brief recovery cup of tea and chat afterwards, all contribute to greater safety and enjoyment.

Session content

At any age, to achieve optimal health related fitness benefits we need to include training in each of the core components of fitness, strength, endurance, flexibility, balance and co-ordination. These need to be combined in a programme that is specific to the purpose, practised regularly, and which progresses at an individualised rate in its frequency, intensity, duration, type and approach. The exercises should use all major muscle groups and should train using each individual's fullest possible, pain-free ranges of movement. Above all, exercise should be enjoyable, accessible, affordable, and educational. It should also encourage a long-term commitment to a more active life. A mix of regular recreational brisk walking and swimming combined with specific exercises to improve strength and flexibility will be effective for most older people. Specific additional aims of a programme for older participants are set out in Box 2.

Further adaptations for vulnerable older patients

With the oldest old and with vulnerable older patients there is a particular emphasis on activities of daily living and enabling maximal independence.[1] The exercise programme, whilst aiming high, must

---

Box 2
The components of an exercise programme for any older person

All of the basic components, viz:

- ► Strength
- ► Endurance
- ► Flexibility
- ► Balance
- ► Coordination

Plus specific, targeted aims, such as:	**All of these plus support strategies such as:**
► Bone loading for wrists, spine and hips	► Home based options
► Functional, postural and pelvic floor muscles	► Telephone support
	► More use of touch
► Dynamic balance, co-ordination and reaction time	► Opportunities for socialisation
► Functional activities (eg sit to stand, get up and down from floor)	► 'Buddy' systems
	► Peer, mentor and befriender schemes
► Correction of localised weakness, asymmetry etc.	► Holistic education programme
► Seated and standing options for all exercises	► Registers and follow up
	► Qualified Exercise for the Older Person Advanced
► Condition-specific sessions	Instructors

---

reflect this, with its primary focus on regaining and maintaining functional mobility.

A combination of chair based mobility, strengthening and stretching exercises that target functional, postural and locomotor muscles, plus simple standing assisted walking and ball games are a sound starting point. Only when progress allows, is supported dynamic balance work introduced.

The type and combinations of exercise must reflect its purpose and the evidence base. For example, programmes designed to improve postural stability must include sustained 3-dimensional movement (eg *Tai chi*), specific dynamic balance and resistance training, and practice of functional floor skills. Accident prevention education, specific home exercise programmes and participant feedback complete the evidence-based, exercise-related guidelines on reducing the risk of falls.[15,16] In dementia care, on the other hand, the focus must be on stimulation, interaction and mobility.[17,18]

To relate the session closely to life for the vulnerable older patient, the exercise activities must provide opportunities for supervised practice of customary activities. Correct techniques for efficient transfers in and out of chairs, beds and cars, taking jumpers on and off, performing a range of towelling actions, picking objects up from the floor, reaching up whilst balancing on the toes, walking and negotiating obstacles and, as soon as safety and skill permits, getting up and down from the floor and even crawling and rolling should be specifically taught and discussed. This demands specialist teaching skills.[16]

Physical support should be progressively decreased whilst ensuring that each individual is allowed to progress at his/her own pace. The fear of a fall or an injury can often be a significant barrier and vulnerable older patients usually need considerable support and encouragement. There should be specific feedback about goals achieved, especially in areas of personal interest to each patient. There should be discreet and effective responses to individual fluctuations in health and energy. A sensitive, skilful exercise practitioner may be the most important part of the programme.[4]

With patients who cannot leave their chair, the aim should be to provide a tailored adaptation of every exercise. Similarly, where movement is not possible, or is inadvisable for a particular body part, an alternative exercise should be provided so that the patient is engaged throughout. Being frequently asked to miss an exercise while others are active can be demotivating.

Dedication and self-motivation are needed when working with patients who need twenty-four hour care. For many patients with dementia, progress is slow and recognition of achievement not always possible. Patience and a high staff to patient ratio are essential to improve participation. Although many of the activities recommended earlier can be adapted easily, staff training is essential. Simple ball games with safe throwing and catching techniques, carefully controlled partner work with resistance bands, music and dancing appear to be greatly enjoyed. Interactive strategies such as asking questions and using specific objects in the room as reference points all assist in sustaining concentration. When successful, these sessions often have quite a party atmosphere.

Subtle cognitive changes can mean that many older participants have greater difficulty remembering techniques, circuit formats or step patterns. Breaking down movement activities into small stages, practising them at slower speeds and rehearsing them each week all assist safety.

Hearing and vision are often impaired in older patients. Briefer, more concise instructions and questions, more frequent repetition, speaking more distinctly with lips clearly visible, and conversing at eye level with the patient can all improve communication and understanding.

Endurance training

Exercise intensity increases the risk of cardiovascular and musculo-skeletal injuries.[4] With all older participants it is important to control the intensity of endurance activities to avoid excessive demand on the myocardium, with its associated risks of ischaemia and rate-related arrhythmias. An adequate warm up is also important (as discussed earlier).

The selection and combination of activities can affect intensity. With regard to walking and cycling, for example, the intensity is relatively constant from one individual to another, whereas in skipping, rebounding, dancing and exercising to music there is much greater variation. A carefully designed session can alternate between brisk and moderate phases, enabling participants to continue exercising for longer, but with greater safety and comfort.

Further adaptations for vulnerable older patients

Initially, endurance training for frailer, older participants may take the form of chair marching (ie a 'marching' action while seated, using first the legs before resting them while the arms take over the marching action). As skill and tolerance increase, arms and legs can 'march' simultaneously. Participants may then progress to a mixture of seated and standing activities (holding the chair), and finally to options performed standing near, but not holding, the chair.

Resistance training

Several studies have demonstrated that appropriate training will improve strength.[1] Most older people will benefit safely by performing a single set of 8–15 repetitions to fatigue of each of 8–10 exercises, twice or three times a week.[19] However, strength gains will transfer most effectively to improved performance of everyday activities only if the practice of these specific functional skills is included in the training.[20] Exercise programmes for all older participants should therefore include not only the core fitness training components but also the practice of functional skills. With vulnerable, older patients, just using body weight is often a sufficient training stimulus. Exercise intensity can be altered by adjustments of the performance of these customary activities (eg by reducing the use of the arms in rising from a chair to increase the intensity of strength training of the lower limb extensors).

There is no evidence that static contractions lasting 5–10 seconds increase the risk of a clinical event in older people.[4] Nevertheless, because of the rapid rises in systolic and diastolic blood pressure, it is usually recommended that older people (especially those with hypertension, coronary artery disease or peripheral vascular disease) avoid high intensity isometric efforts lasting more than about 5 seconds.

In all weight training activities the participant must understand the importance of avoiding the problems of the Valsalva manoeuvre (straining against a closed glottis).

Further adaptations for vulnerable older patients

Some patients, especially those with arthritis, may have to use lighter weights (with a higher number of repetitions) and limit the range of movement for some exercises.[19] Progression may have to be particularly cautious.

Just as with endurance training (see above) strength training may have to be broken down into shorter, more frequent episodes. Functional, chair-based arm, wrist and leg extensor exercises performed after bathing and dressing, and repeated before dinner, appear to be a realistic goal in several of our ward settings. This 'exercise snack' approach is also used in the self-directed, home-based sessions, which supplement our weekly, supervised community sessions for frailer older patients. If longer bouts of resistance exercise are used, longer recovery periods are needed before the next session to reduce the risk of pain and to enhance performance.[4,21]

Amongst frailer older participants, counting out loud appears to work well to prevent a Valsalva effect and is usually preferable to the more specific technique of 'breathing out on the effort'. Amongst those with short-term memory problems the latter can result in confusion, anxiety and unnecessary risk.

With the frailest patients a less direct approach may be called for in the 'wooing phase'. Here, resistance training can be achieved through a range of musculo-skeletal activities presented in fun, flexible, imaginative formats. The colours, movement and group activity involved in lifting and lowering a parachute often elicit enthusiastic participation and enable the exercise practitioner to engage the group whilst still aiming for the requisite number of lifts. Further resistance can be added by increasing the height of the lift or by introducing a weighted ball into the centre of the parachute.

Preventing injuries

Injury prevention is a high priority. Even stiffness and minor overuse injuries reduce enjoyment, may affect compliance and can often be avoided. The design of the session, the supervision and monitoring of performance together with education and guidance of participants can substantially reduce hazards.

Overuse injuries, or 'too much too soon' injuries, occur during participation in both endurance and strength training programmes and are not uncommon amongst older participants.[22–4] As with cardiovascular risk, exercise intensity is a major contributor. To reduce the risk of exacerbating an existing joint condition, the load on joints, bones and other support structures can be controlled by ensuring biomechanically sound positions, correct alignment and correct technique.

Precise, audible teaching instructions and visible, skilled demonstrations together with good observation of the participants are essential to ensure safety. Also important are non-slip floor surfaces, sturdy chairs, adequate lighting, handrails and uncluttered entrances, corridors and exercise areas.[3]

Further adaptations for vulnerable older patients

Patients with osteoporosis should avoid sit-ups and other exercises which cause spinal loading in flexion.[25] All older patients with muscle weakness, particularly those with a history of joint, muscle or connective tissue damage caused by previous injury, overuse or disease, should use an especially cautious training load initially, with predominantly isometric work at first, then progress to light isotonic work. The emphasis is on control throughout the range of movement, careful monitoring, progression in very small increments and patient feedback.

One of the most significant potential benefits of exercise for vulnerable older patients is a reduction in the risk of falls.[26,27] However, without sufficient care, some older people may suffer more falls because participation increases their exposure to risk.[28] Thorough preparation of frail participants, especially those with a history of falls, ensures adequate strength, endurance, co-ordination and flexibility before they embark on unsupported dynamic balance work. Moreover, the exercises must not include any movements with a high risk of falling. For example, there must be no turns of more than 90° nor any exercises which involve lateral movement of one leg across the other.[15]

Wearing hip protectors greatly reduces the risk of hip fracture in a fall[29] and also improves self-efficacy.[30] The use of these is strongly recommended, especially in specialist fall prevention sessions. Compliance may be improved if the instructor also wears hip protectors.[15]

Orthostatic hypotension may be a significant problem. Particular care needs to be taken on rising after lying on the floor. Mat work activities such as rolling, crawling and ankle strengthening exercises, are ways of ensuring an intermediate position between lying and standing. Such activities also give practice in important coping strategies that the patient can use to rise again in the event of a fall. This also appears to reduce fear of falling.[31] Being ready to steady the patient for a few seconds after standing until equilibrium is restored must be standard exercise practice with this group.

Working in pairs (with resistance bands, for example) whilst fun and interactive, must be delayed until strict form and awareness of each other's abilities are established.

The duration of exercise sessions can play a role in injury. Shorter bouts of endurance or resistance training performed more frequently, even several times a day, are less fatiguing and so may be less likely to predispose to injuries than longer bouts performed less often.[4]

Long-term programming

The aim is long-term commitment to a mixture of activities. This might include walking, swimming, weight-, circuit-, and step-training, exercise to music, dancing, chair work, *Tai chi*, golf and bowls. With regard to more vulnerable older patients it may be that bowls and weight training are executed whilst seated, *Tai chi* performed initially from a static base, and walking done between parallel bars. With circuit training it may be best for the patients to remain seated while the exercise practitioner changes the circuit cards. Provision must cater for a wide range of disabilities and initial levels of physical activity.

Long-term adherence is enhanced if the programme provides regular opportunities for socialisation. A suitably equipped area should be identified so that participants can rest and chat comfortably and safely before and after sessions. In addition participants should be involved in planning, selecting and evaluating the programme. A recent 'Fit Folk Talks' series, evolved with our patients, has been highly popular.

The use of appropriate equipment, an accessible venue, an elder-friendly environment, and a recreational approach (eg incorporating music and games) increases enjoyment, confidence and commitment.

Scheduling is extremely important. Year round programming for older participants requires flexibility and resourcefulness to respond to changes in the weather and temperature, which in turn affect footwear and clothing selections.

Further adaptations for vulnerable older patients

In care settings, consultation with staff and patients helps to ensure that the timing of sessions is realistic and that, where appropriate, sessions can be supported by staff allocated to specific roles (such as assisting individual patients). Care staff who are interested in leading groups can undertake further training.

In addition a telephone call to care staff 45 minutes prior to each session is helpful and ensures that patients are mentally prepared, ready to go, appropriately dressed and alert, and that staff are on hand and aware. For their part the exercise practitioner needs to ensure that all sessions keep strictly to time and that all equipment is set out and cleared away safely. Regular feedback to the rest of the interdisciplinary care team on each patient's progress is particularly important so that activity and exercise become integrated into the care plan.

Transition to a community setting

A short, tailored induction period to precede the transition from a healthcare setting to a community recreational exercise setting has been shown to be effective in increasing long term adherence in cardiac rehabilitation patients[32] and we find it works well for vulnerable older patients in both secondary and primary care. The induction phase (8–10 weeks) enables the acquisition of basic exercise techniques and discussion about any personal concerns and problems. It establishes friendships with other group members and with the exercise practitioner. This phase may be held in the hospital, in residential care, in general practice, or in the patient's home.

The transition itself is given considerable attention. For the first two weeks of the transition the exercise practitioner, the general practice staff, the recreation club staff and even the patient transport staff are all on hand to direct, assist and welcome patients until everyone has settled into the new regimen. This approach helps to reduce the attrition that often results from practical difficulties due to transport and anxiety about unfamiliar surroundings and people. Patients are supported by telephone contact during the induction and transition phases and any absences are followed up. Registers are kept at all sessions and strong links are kept between the healthcare and recreational settings so that patients have a sense of continuity and so that medical re-referral, if needed, can occur easily. The 'route' for each patient is individual. Although most go directly to the community setting from the induction group, several may remain as founder members of the next induction group until such time as they are able and willing to make the transition. This individualised approach to programming for vulnerable older patients has catered for secondary and primary care patients with a wide range of pathologies and disabilities, including patients with chronic and late onset mental health problems. It is currently being implemented in practices throughout north London.

Re-referral back to the clinical setting

Detection of a new or worsened condition is an indication for the exercise practitioner to refer the patient back to the referring clinical setting until such time as inclusion becomes appropriate again.

Education

It is important to inform participants about the early recognition of significant symptoms (see *The role of the doctor*). Knowing there is a difference between pain and discomfort and that 'where there is pain and strain there is no gain' are welcome and often entirely new messages for older participants. Other important messages can be communicated in a positive way by the exercise practitioner in the pre-exercise assessment and reinforced during sessions. These include specific physical pointers as to when exercise should be stopped and when it should continue. It is also useful to emphasise the importance of:

▌ warming-up and warming-down
▌ resting before and after the activity
▌ working at one's own level and adjusting activities or intensity on days when 'energy' is low
▌ not exercising when feeling unwell.

Combining these safety messages with motivating information, about the purpose of each exercise and the benefits of different types of exercise, assists the older person in making more informed activity choices and in taking responsibility for their safety and comfort during exercise.

Patients can be trained to 'listen to their body', using a scale for the Rating of Perceived Exertion (RPE).[33] This gives the patient a useful measure of effort during endurance and strength activities. Also, where relevant, there is a pain scale[33] for those whose chronic pain may be influenced by exercise and a dyspnoea scale[34] for those in whom breathlessness is a prominent symptom. Whatever method is used to monitor intensity, close observation by the exercise practitioner of each participant during each exercise remains important.

Instructors should give written information to both patients and health professionals that includes guidelines on exercise for the older person, the contraindications to activity participation, the benefits, aims, level, structure and content of the session, self monitoring and exercise technique tips, signs when exercise can continue and when it should be stopped, when to seek medical advice, costs and, finally, the qualifications and experience of the instructor.

Specialised qualifications and training

The skills required to ensure optimal performance, safety and enjoyment for older participants are important and specialised.[3,35,36] Competence to plan and deliver such programmes implies both theoretical knowledge and practical experience in selecting, adapting and supervising safe, appropriate exercise in ways that accommodate the heterogeneity of older people. Qualifications now exist in this specialised area and exercise instructors should be able to demonstrate that they are properly trained. It is recommended that health professionals refer older people only to exercise professionals with appropriate specialist qualifications and on the Professional Register for Exercise and Fitness (England) or its equivalent elsewhere in the UK.[37]

Conclusion

Exercise has an important place in a holistic approach to health management, yet its potential for the vulnerable older patient is often underestimated and under-utilised. Improvements in functional strength and mobility can be achieved even in frail patients in their ninth decade. Improvements can still occur in older people who have a variety of disabilities, including those who are unable to walk or stand. Even seemingly trivial absolute levels of activity may be expected to contribute to the restoration or maintenance of endurance, strength, flexibility and balance in old age. Small increases in these components of fitness can lead to large improvements in the quality of life. Critical to the safety and effectiveness of these programmes is the informed collaboration of health professionals with exercise practitioners who have acquired the necessary, specialised programming and teaching skills. In this way, the considerable potential benefits of physical activity can be enjoyed by even the most vulnerable elderly patient.

Acknowledgements

I am grateful to Dr Dawn Skelton and Dr Katie Malbut-Shennan for helpful comments on the draft typescript and to Professor Archie Young for his editorial influence and expertise. I am grateful to Professor Paul Wallace and Dr Steve Iliffe at the Department of Primary Care and Population Sciences at the Royal Free and University College School of Medicine, the Hampstead Group Practice and Camden Leisure Services for allowing me to include information on the Primary Care Project For Older People in Camden and to the Old Age Psychiatry Department at the Royal Free Hospital for the inclusion of information regarding in-service programmes.

References

1   Young A. The health benefits of physical activity for a healthier old age. In: Young A, Harries M (eds). *Physical Activity for Patients: An Exercise Prescription.* London: Royal College of Physicians of London, 2001.

2   Mazzeo RS, Cavanagh P, Evans WJ, *et al.* Exercise and physical activity for older adults. *Medicine and Science in Sports and Exercise.* 2000; **30(6)**: 992–1008.

3   Young A, Dinan S. Active in later life. In: McLatchie G, Harries M, Williams C, King J (eds). *ABC of Sports Medicine (2nd edition).* London: BMJ Books. 2000.

4   Haskell WL. Medical clearance for exercise program participation by older persons: The clinical versus the public health approach. In: Huber G (ed). *Healthy Aging, Activity and Sports.* Gamburg: Health Promotion Publications, 1997.

5   Durstine JL, Bloomquist LE, Figoni SF, *et al* (eds). *ACSM's Exercise Management for Persons with Chronic Diseases and Disabilities.* Champaign, Illinois: Human Kinetics,1997.

6   Dinan S, Messent P. Guidelines: promoting physical activity with people with disabilities. London: Health Education Authority; 1997.

7   Heath GW, Fentem PH. Physical activity among persons with disabilities – a public health perspective. *Exercise and Sports Sciences Reviews* 1997; **25**: 195–234.

8   Department of Health. *Exercise Referral Systems: A National Quality Assurance Framework.* London: The Stationery Office, 2001.

9   Young A, Bös K. Assessment for physical activity in old age. Introduction. In: Huber G (ed). *Healthy Aging, Activity and Sports.* Gamburg: Health Promotion Publications 1997.

10 Rikli RE, Jones CJ. Development and validation of a functional fitness test for community-residing older adults. *Journal of Aging and Physical Activity* 1999; **7**: 129–61.

11 Gill TM, Di Pietro L, Krumholz HM. Role of exercise stress testing and safety monitoring for older persons starting an exercise program. *Journal of the American Medical Association* 2000; **284(3)**: 342–9.

12 Shephard RJ. Benefits of sport and physical activity for the disabled: implications for the individual and for society. *Scand J Rehabilitation Med* 1991; **23**: 51–9.

13 DeBusk RF, Stenestrand U, Sheehan M, Haskell WL. Training effects of long versus short bouts of exercise in healthy subjects. *American Journal of Cardiology* 1990; **65**: 1010–13.

14 Ebisu T. Splitting the distance of endurance running. On cardiovascular endurance and blood lipids. *Japanese Journal of Physical Education* 1985; **30**: 37–43.

15 Skelton D, Dinan S. Exercise for falls management. *Physiotherapy Theory and Practice* 1999; **15**: 105–20.

16 Dinan S, Skelton D (eds). *Exercise for Improving Postural Stability and Reducing the Risk of Falls and Injuries. A Specialist Training Course for Health and Exercise Professionals.* Leicester: Leicester College, 2000.

17 Dinan S. Fit for life; why exercise is vital for everyone. *Journal of Dementia Care* 1998; **6(3)**: 22–5.

18 Cayton H, Graham N, Warner J. *Alzheimer's at Your Fingertips.* London: Class Publishing, 1997.

19 Feigenbaum MS, Pollock ML. Prescription of resistance training for health and disease. *Medicine and Science in Sports and Exercise* 1998; **31**: 38–45.

20 Skelton DA, McLaughlin AW. Training functional ability in old age. *Physiotherapy* 1996; **82**: 159–67.

21 Ettinger WH, Burns R, Messier SP, *et al.* A randomised trial comparing aerobic exercise and resistance exercise with a health education program in older adults with knee osteoarthritis. *J Amer Med Ass* 1997; **277**: 25–31.

22 Carroll JF, Pollock ML, Graves JE, *et al.* Incidence of injury during moderate- and high-intensity walking training in the elderly. *Journal of Gerontology* 1992; **47**: M61–M66.

23 Pollock ML, Carroll JF, Graves JE, *et al.* Injuries and adherence to walk/jog and resistance training programs in the elderly. *Medicine and Science in Sports and Exercise* 1991; **23**: 1194–200.

24 Pollock ML, Gettman LR, Milesis CA, *et al.* Effects of frequency and duration of training on attrition and incidence of injury. *Medicine and Science in Sports and Exercise* 1977; **9**: 31–6.

25 Sinaki M, Mikkelson BA. Postmenopausal spinal osteoporosis: flexion versus extension exercises. *Archives of Physical Medicine and Rehabilitation* 1984; **65**: 593–6.

26 Tinetti ME, Baker DL, McAvay G, *et al.* A multifactorial intervention to reduce the risk of falling among elderly people living in the community. *N Engl J Med* 1994; **331**: 821–7.

27 Campbell AJ, Robertson MC, Gardner MM, *et al.* Randomised controlled trial of a general practice, home based exercise programme for falls prevention in elderly women. *Brit Med J* 1997; **315**: 1065–9.

28 Ebrahim S, Thompson PW, Baskaran V, Evans K. Randomised placebo-controlled trial of brisk walking in the prevention of postmenopausal osteoporosis. *Age Ageing* 1997; **26**: 253–60.

29 Kannus P, Parkkari J, Niemi S, *et al.* Prevention of hip fracture in elderly people with use of a hip protector. *New England Journal of Medicine* 2000; **343**: 1506–13.

30 Cameron ID, Stafford B, Cumming RG, *et al.* Hip protectors improve falls self-efficacy. *Age and Ageing* 2000; **29**: 57–62.

31 Simpson JM, Marsh N, Harrington R. Managing falls among elderly people. *British Journal of Occupational Therapy* 1998; **61**: 165–8.

32 Bell J, Coats AJ, Hardman AE. Exercise testing and prescription. In: Coats AJ (ed). *British Association of Cardiac Rehabilitation Guidelines.* Oxford: Blackwell Science, 1995.

33 Borg GAV. *Borg's Perceived Exertion and Pain Scales.* Champaign, Ilinois: Human Kinetics. 1998.

34 Burdon JGW, Juniper EF, Killian KJ, *et al.* The perception of breathlessness in asthma. *American Review of Respiratory Disease* 1982; **126**: 825–8.

35 Jones CJ, Rikli RE. Implications for curriculum development and professional preparation in physical education. *Journal of Aging and Physical Activity* 1994; **2**: 261–72.

36 Dinan S, Laventure B. The provision and certification of training in relation to older people and physical activity in the United Kingdom. In: Huber G (ed). *Healthy Aging, Activity and Sports.* Gamburg: Health Promotion Publications 1997.

37 Laventure B. The clinical exercise practitioner. In: Young A, Harries M (eds) *Physical Activity for Patients: An Exercise Prescription.* London: Royal College of Physicians, 2001.

8 | Delivering an exercise prescription for patients with coronary artery disease

Jennifer Bell

Eligibility and risk stratification

Exercise training should be considered part of the routine management of coronary artery disease (CAD) and should be widely available (Box 1). CAD patients for whom exercise is contraindicated are predominantly those with unstable symptoms or conditions (Box 2).

Box 1
Coronary artery disease patients who should have ready access to exercise training:

► Post-myocardial infarction (MI)
► Post-coronary artery bypass graft surgery (CABGS)
► Post-percutaneous transluminal coronary angioplasty (PTCA)
► Post-transplantation
► Congestive heart failure (CHF)
► Stable angina

Box 2
Coronary artery disease patients for whom exercise training is contraindicated:

► Unstable angina
► Resting SBP $\geq$ 200mmHg or DBP $\geq$ 110mmHg
► Uncontrolled tachycardia
► Significant resting ST segment displacement
► Uncontrolled atrial or ventricular arrhythmias
► Uncompensated congestive heart failure
► Recent embolism
► Significant aortic stenosis

Even in patients for whom training is appropriate, exercise carries a risk.[1] Implementing a risk stratification model to classify participants according to their risk of death or cardiovascular complication (based on one year mortality and morbidity data) should, therefore, be standard practice in both clinical and community settings. The American Association of Cardiovascular and Pulmonary Rehabilitation (AACVPR) risk stratification criteria for cardiac patients is shown in Box 3. UK guidelines have also been developed.[3] Exercising higher risk patients is a matter of clinical judgement and would normally be undertaken only in a clinically supervised programme.

The components of exercise prescription

The development of cardiovascular endurance is the primary objective for CAD patients since the training-induced reductions in heart rate and blood pressure at reference submaximal workloads reduce myocardial oxygen demand and thereby delay the onset of ischaemia and lessen the potential for arrhythmias. Endurance exercise is defined as any activity which uses large muscle groups, can be maintained for a prolonged period and is rhythmic and aerobic in nature. The inclusion of a variety of training modes within the individual prescription or the class format will minimize the incidence of over-use injuries, maximise peripheral adaptation (as for example when activities which require a contribution from both upper and lower body musculature are included) and will increase patient motivation and adherence. Nevertheless, walking remains the mainstay of exercise prescription for cardiac patients, particularly in the early stages of recovery and when activity is unsupervised, either as part of home-based programmes[4,5] or between supervised sessions. An incremental walking programme typical of those prescribed for patients on discharge from hospital is presented in Table 1. The duration of walks throughout the week can be varied but an average of 10 miles per week is known to be associated with positive health gains. Patients should be advised to:

▮ walk at a pace which feels comfortable and to start and finish the walk at a slower pace

▮ make a note of how they feel after each day's walk and, if tired for some time after completing the walk, they should reduce the distance or the speed the following day

▮ stop if any chest pain is experienced (use Glyceryl Trinitrate (GTN) if it has been prescribed) and wait until the pain goes before continuing at a reduced pace. If the frequency or severity of chest

Box 3
American Association of Cardiovascular and Pulmonary Rehabilitation (AACVPR) risk stratification criteria for cardiac patients:[2]

Lowest Risk

▸ No significant LV dysfunction (EF>50%)
▸ No resting or exercise-induced complex dysrhythmias
▸ Uncomplicated MI; CABG; angioplasty, atherectomy, or stent;
  – absence of CHF or signs/symptoms indicating post-event ischaemia
▸ Normal hemodynamics with exercise or recovery
▸ Asymptomatic including absence of angina with exertion or recovery
▸ Functional capacity ≥7.0 METS*
▸ Absence of clinical depression

Lowest risk classification is assumed when each of the risk factors in the category is present.

Moderate risk

▸ Moderately impaired left ventricular function (EF = 40–49%)
▸ Signs/symptoms including angina at moderate levels of exercise (5–6.9 METs) or in recovery

Moderate risk is assumed for patients who do not meet the classification of either highest risk or lowest risk.

High risk

▸ Decreased LV function (EF < 40%)
▸ Survivor of cardiac arrest or sudden death
▸ Complex ventricular dysrhythmia at rest or with exercise
▸ MI or cardiac surgery complicated by cardiogenic shock, CHF, and/or signs/symptoms of post-procedure ischaemia
▸ Abnormal hemodynamics with exercise (especially flat or decreasing systolic blood pressure or chronotropic incompetence with increasing workload)
▸ Signs/symptoms including angina pectoris at low levels of exercise (< 5.0 METS) or in recovery
▸ Functional capacity < 5.0 METS*
▸ Clinically significant depression

Highest risk classification is assumed with the presence of any one of the risk factors included in this category.

*NOTE: If measured functional capacity is not available, this variable is not considered in the risk-stratification process.

LV = left ventricular;
MI = myocardial infarction;
CABG = coronary artery bypass graft;

CHF = congestive heart failure;
MET = metabolic equivalent;
EF = ejection fraction.

Table 1. Walking guidelines for cardiac patients.

Week	RPE (Borg scale)	Duration (min)	Distance (yds)	Frequency (per day)
1	9–11	5	200	1–2
2	9–11	10	400–500	2
3	9–11	15	500–750	2
4	11–12	20	750–1,250	1–2
5	11–12	20–30	1,250–1,750	1–2
6	11–12	30–40	1,750–3,000	1–2
Thereafter, an average of 1.5–2 miles per day at a pace that represents an RPE of 11–12				

RPE= Rating of perceived exertion on the Borg scale.[6]

    pain increases or it is provoked at slower walking speeds, the GP should be consulted

▌ wait 40–50 min after a main meal before starting their walk

▌ avoid walking in extremes of temperature, ie very hot or humid or very cold or windy.

There appears to be a gradation in the benefits conferred. It is well documented that CAD patients who expend about 250–300kcals per session and 1,000–1,500 kcals per week in additional physical activity will improve their aerobic capacity by 15–30% over a 4–6 month period.[7] There is some evidence that a minimum of 1,600 kcal per week may halt the progression of CAD and atherosclerotic regression may be achieved with a weekly energy expenditure of about 2,200 kcal.[8]

Within the recommended ranges of Frequency, Intensity and Time (or duration) (FIT) of training (Table 2) similar conditioning effects can be expected from any programme which realises comparable weekly energy expenditure. Consequently the FIT components may be adjusted to provide an optimal prescription for individuals of varying cardiovascular and general medical status. For example, an individual who has a peak exercise capacity of 6 METs (6 times resting energy expenditure) is exercising at only 50% of his capacity when walking at 2.5mph (equivalent to 3 METs) and, assuming a weight of about 75kg will need to walk for just over 4 hours per week to expend 1,000kcals. A patient with a peak capacity of 4 METs would be exercising at 75% of his capacity when walking at 2.5 mph but can achieve the same total energy expenditure by offsetting a reduction in speed with an increase in the duration and/or frequency of walking.[9]

Table 2. The FIT principle (Adapted from the BACR Phase IV Exercise Instructor Training Manual, 2000[11]).

	Programme Clinical Phase III	Community based Phase IV (patients who achieve 5 METs)
Frequency	2–3 per week (eg 1–2 rehabilitation classes + 1–2 home sessions, other days – walk or leisure activities)	3 per week
Intensity		
Maximal heart rate (%)	60–75	60–80
$\dot{V}O_2$ peak (%)	~40–60	~40–70
RPE [Borg scale]	12–13	13–15
Time (min)	20–30	30–60
Type		
Supervised	Any cardiovascular activity (commonly gym-based or circuits)	Any endurance activities (excluding competitive sport)
Independent	Walking, cycling, home-based circuit	Any endurance activities (excluding competitive sport)

Intensity

This issue is critical because vigorous activity carries a greatly increased risk of precipitating adverse events such as myocardial infarction (MI) or arrhythmias.[1] Frequent, moderate intensity exercise is recommended for CAD patients since it will optimise benefits without increasing the risk of adverse events.[10] For individuals with very diminished functional capacity, several short bouts of exercise (as little as 5–10 min) throughout the day at ~40–50% of $\dot{V}O_2$ peak may be advisable.[12]

Ideally, training heart rate (Table 2) is based on information derived from a maximal or symptom-limited exercise ECG test but such information is often not available to health professionals or exercise instructors. In the absence of maximal test data or if, for diagnostic purposes, a patient performs the exercise test 'off medication', other methods for establishing appropriate training intensity have to be used. Age-adjusted predicted maximal rates can be used (220 bpm minus age in years is one formula), but some individuals will have an actual maximal heart rate 20bpm higher or lower than that predicted. Consequently, predicted maximal heart rates should be used only in conjunction with a rating of perceived exertion (RPE)[6] (Box 4). This scale is accepted as a valid and reproducible indicator of the intensity of steady-state exercise and is also used for monitoring exercise intensity in patients whose medication blunts their heart rate response, for example, those taking β-blockers and some calcium channel blockers.

The intensity of exercise may also be regulated by choosing activities according to their known MET (metabolic equivalent) values (Table 3). If an individual assesses walking at 3 mph as 12–13 on the Borg RPE scale (corresponding to 60% of $\dot{V}O_2$ max), then activities of comparable MET value can be prescribed in the knowledge that they will present an

---

Box 4
Borg Scale of rating of perceived exertion

6	No exertion at all	15	Hard (heavy)
7		16	
8	Extremely light	17	Very hard
9	Very light	18	
10		19	Extremely hard
11	Light	20	Maximal exertion
12			
13	Somewhat hard		
14			

Table 3. Appropriate MET values for various activities (Adapted from ACSM, 1995).[13]

Activity	MET value	Activity	MET value
Walking		Swimming	
at 2 mph	2.5	Breast stroke	8–9
at 2.5 mph	2.9	Freestyle	9–10
at 3 mph	3.3		
at 3.75	3.9	Tennis	4–9
Cycling		Skipping	
at 5 mph	2–3	60–80 rpm	8–10
at 10 mph	5–6	120–140 rpm	11–12
at 13 mph	8–9	Stepping (using 12″ (30cm) step	
Dancing		Rate of stepping (cycles per min):	
Ballroom	4–6	16	5
Aerobic dance class	6–9	24	7.5
		32	10

equivalent training stimulus. Knowledge of MET values is also important to exclude activities that might pose a risk to certain individuals. Skipping (8–12 METs) or freestyle swimming (9–10 METs), for example, would be entirely inappropriate advice for someone with a peak capacity of 7 METs. Table 3 shows that some activities have a wide range of MET values, while others do not. The MET value of some activities is relatively constant between individuals, mainly because there is little variation in individual execution. For example, there is very little difference in the way individuals walk or cycle. In contrast, there can be great variation in the way 'free-moving' activities such as dancing, skipping or rebounding on a mini-trampoline are executed. Precise control of the exercise prescription is necessary for cardiac patients (particularly in early recovery post event and for those with stable angina). Therefore, activities which can be maintained at prescribed workrates and which permit uniform modification (eg by altering the speed of walking or the resistance on a cycle ergometer) are preferred to those that are not amenable to standardised prescription.

Whatever the objective method used for monitoring intensity, it is important to observe individuals for excessive breathlessness, loss of quality of movement, unusual pallor or excessive sweating, all of which are inappropriate responses to a moderate level of exertion.

The exercise programme

Warm-up

Preparation for activity in older adults and especially in those with cardiac disease must be more gradual than with younger, healthy individuals. Fifteen minutes of preparation is recommended.[12] A gradual increase in the size and range of movements performed will delay the onset of ischaemia by allowing adequate time for coronary blood flow to increase to meet the greater myocardial demand. Gradual increments in myocardial workload will also lessen the risk of arrhythmias, which can be a consequence of abrupt increases in demand and concomitant elevated sympathetic activity. As a guideline, individuals should be within 20 bpm of their prescribed training heart rate at the end of the warm-up or, if RPE is used in place of heart rate monitoring, a rating no higher than 10–11 on the original scale.[6]

Cardiovascular conditioning

The type of activity used for conditioning may adopt a continuous or an interval approach. Continuous training, as the name implies, involves uninterrupted activity usually performed at a constant submaximal intensity. Its advantage is the ease with which intensity may be prescribed and monitored. Walking, jogging, cycling, rowing, bench stepping and swimming all lend themselves to a continuous approach. Interval training entails bouts of relatively intensive work separated by periods of rest or less intensive activity. Its main advantage is that the total volume of work accomplished is greater than when the same intensity of exercise is continuous; consequently the stimulus to physiological change is greater. The transition from one activity to another also provides a time for social interaction and support which probably aid long-term compliance.

In clinically supervised programmes, interval style circuit training is the favoured format for rehabilitation classes. Participants spend a fixed time (ranging from 30 seconds to 2 min) at 'cardiovascular (CV) stations' and either rest or perform a lower intensity activity before moving on to the next CV station. The lower intensity or 'active recovery' stations are usually designed to increase the endurance of specific muscle groups (eg triceps, pectorals, trapezius) used in activities of daily living.

Individualisation of the cardiovascular component of the programme is achieved through variation in the:

▌ duration at each CV station*

▌ intensity* (by changing the resistance or the speed or range of movement)

▌ period of rest between stations

▌ overall duration of conditioning.
   (* In general the duration of activity is extended before increasing the intensity.)

Exercises involving a recumbent position are discouraged within the circuit because:

▌ some older participants have difficulty in getting up and down

▌ following vigorous activity, the increase in venous return on lying down enhances pre-load and thereby myocardial workload which increases the risk of arrhythmias and angina in some individuals

▌ there is an increased risk of orthostatic hypotension.

Any recumbent work (eg for the abdominals or erector spinae) should be performed *after* completion of the circuit and a cool-down period.

On transition to community-based programmes patients are encouraged to progress by extending the duration of their cardiovascular sessions and to use a more continuous training approach. Many patients will benefit from gym-based CV programmes and for some resistance training may be appropriate.

Resistance training

In the past, training to increase strength (as opposed to endurance) was considered to be inappropriate for individuals with established heart disease. This was because the increase in intrathoracic pressure associated with resistance training results in an increase in myocardial workload mainly due to the rise in arterial blood pressure. Some early studies suggested that the isometric component caused a reduced ejection fraction, left ventricle wall motion abnormalities and an increased incidence of arrhythmias. More recent studies[14,15] have generally reported that cardiovascular and haemodynamic responses to resistance training in CAD patients and in normal subjects are similar and, because of increased diastolic pressure, may even enhance myocardial perfusion. However, in the UK, it remains unusual to incorporate strength training into clinically supervised programmes unless it is indicated for vocational reasons.

In the absence of further research, guidelines remain relatively conservative; two sets, each of eight to ten exercises involving the major muscle groups, performed at least twice a week, is the usual recommendation. The American College of Sports Medicine (ACSM) advocates just a single set (comprising 10–12 repetitions which can be performed 'comfortably'), of each of up to 10–12 exercises.[16] This is based on evidence that strength gains derived from one set are similar to those when several sets are performed, and adherence to less time-consuming programmes is better. The contraindications to resistance training are unsurprising (Box 5).

Box 5
Contraindications for resistance training:

▶ Abnormal haemodynamic responses with exercise
▶ Ischaemic changes during graded exercise testing
▶ Poor left ventricular function
▶ Uncontrolled hypertension or arrhythmias
▶ Exercise capacity less than 6 METs

Cool-down component

A period of 10 min is recommended for cool-down at the end of the cardiovascular component. The cool-down should incorporate movements of diminishing intensity and passive stretching of the major muscle groups used during the conditioning phase. In addition, patients should be observed for up to 30 min after the exercise session. This period of gentle activity and subsequent observation are important because:

▋ there is an increased risk of hypotension in this group. For some this is a specific side-effect of their medication. In addition, there is an age-related slowing of baroreceptor responsiveness which increases the risk of venous pooling following sustained exercise

▋ in older adults heart rates take longer to return to pre-exercise rates

▋ raised sympathetic activity during vigorous exercise increases the risk of arrhythmias during the immediate period following cessation of exercise.

Progression

The duration, frequency or intensity of training can be increased in order to maintain the training stimulus. Ideally, serial exercise testing will form the basis on which the prescription is modified in order to ensure that it continues safely to provoke physiological adaptation. In the absence of exercise testing, heart rate monitoring and rating of perceived exertion at reference workloads may be used to establish the appropriateness of increasing any of the three variables, either singly or in combination with one another. The way in which exercise prescription is progressed and the rate at which it is progressed will be highly variable between individuals with CAD, and will be a function of many factors including age, severity of disease, motivation, dual pathology and compliance.

References

1   Willich SN, Lewis M, Lowel H, *et al.* Physical exertion as a trigger of acute myocardial infarction. *N Engl J Med* 1993; **329**: 1684–90.

2   American Association of Cardiovascular and Pulmonary Rehabilitation (AACVPR). *Guidelines for Cardiac Rehabilitation and Secondary Prevention Program (3e).* Champaign, Illinois: Human Kinetics, 1999.

3   Tipson R. The exercise component of cardiac rehabilitation. *Br J Ther Rehab* 1997; **4(6)**: 317.

4   Lewin B, Robertson IH, Cay EL, *et al.* Effects of self-help post myocardial infarction rehabilitation on psychological adjustment and use of health services. *Lancet* 1992; **339**: 1036–40.

5   Dressendorfer RH, Franklin BA, Cameron JL, *et al.* Exercise training frequency in early post-infarction cardiac rehabilitation. Influence on aerobic conditioning. *J Cardiolpulmonary Rehab* 1995; **15**: 269–76.

6   Borg GA. *Borg's Perceived Exertion and Pain Scales.* Champaign: Illinois: Human Kinetics, 1998.

7   Balady GJ, Fletcher BJ, Froelicher ES, *et al.* Cardiac rehabilitation programs. A statement for healthcare professionals from the American Heart Association. *Circulation* 1994; **90**: 1602–10.

8   Hambrecht R, Niebauer J, Marburger C, *et al.* Various intensities of leisure time physical activity in patients with coronary artery disease: effects on cardiorespiratory fitness and progression of coronary artherosclerotic lesions. *J Cardiopulmonary Rehab* 1994; **14**: 197–8.

9   Wenger NK. Rehabilitation of the coronary patient: a preview of tomorrow. *J Cardiopulmonary Rehab* 1991; **11**: 93–8.

10 Dafoe W, Huston P. Current trends in cardiac rehabilitation. *Can Med Ass J* 1997; **156**: 527–32.

11 Bell J (ed). *Phase IV Exercise Instructor Training Manual (2e).* London: British Association for Cardiac Rehabilitation, 2000.

12 Bell J, Coats AJ, Hardman AE. Exercise testing and prescription. In: Coats AJ (ed). *BACR Guidelines for Cardiac Rehabilitation.* Oxford: Blackwell Science, 1995.

13 American College of Sports Medicine (ACSM). *Guidelines for Exercise Testing and Prescription (5e).* London: Williams and Wilkins, 1995.

14 Squires RW, Muri AJ, Anderson LJ, *et al.* Weight training during Phase II (early outpatient) cardiac rehabilitation: Heart rate and blood pressure responses. *J Cardiac Rehab* 1991; **11**: 360–4.

15 Williams MA. *Exercise Testing and Training in the Elderly Cardiac Patient.* Champaign, Illinois: Human Kinetics, 1994.

16 American College of Sports Medicine (ACSM). Position stand – exercise for patients with coronary artery disease. *Med Sci Sport Exerc* 1994; **26**: I–IV.

9 | Delivering an exercise prescription for patients with chronic obstructive pulmonary disease

Christopher J Clark, David Sword and Lorna M Cochrane

Introduction

There is strong evidence that exercise programmes can reduce disability in patients with chronic respiratory disease, particularly when conducted within multidisciplinary programmes of pulmonary rehabilitation.[1–3] Chronic obstructive pulmonary disease (COPD) is a major cause of disability in the UK, but patients can nevertheless achieve considerable benefit in terms of reduced dyspnoea, improved mobility, improved performance of activities of daily living and improved sense of mastery, by rehabilitation which systematically identifies each patient's needs and individualises their exercise prescription accordingly. The process by which this is achieved involves:

▌ clear characterisation of the patient in terms of mental and physical health, attitudes, and illness severity

▌ provision of a range of programme options

▌ the use of one or more evaluation instruments to monitor progress.

The main symptom of many patients with COPD is breathlessness on exertion. The three main underlying mechanisms are listed in Box 1.

Exercise limitation may be predominantly due to symptoms other than breathlessness, such as leg fatigue, in more than 30% of patients.[4] This is because of peripheral muscle weakness,[5] which is presumably secondary to inactivity. The disuse atrophy may also be aggravated by chronic hypoxaemia and poor nutritional status. Thus a vicious cycle begins in which secondary deconditioning may have an undue impact, reducing mobility to the point where the patient may simply lose the ability to exercise vigorously enough to be limited by breathlessness. Cardiopulmonary exercise testing is used to evaluate the factors causing breathlessness and exercise limitation in patients with chronic lung disease, both in specialist centres and in lung function laboratories in district general hospitals. Alternative 'field' methods such as timed walk tests[6] or shuttle tests[7] can also be very helpful where there is less access to

Box 1
Main mechanisms underlying breathlessness

▶ A reduction in maximal ventilatory capacity – ie reduced breathing reserve – due to narrowed airways causing increased resistance to flow
▶ An increased ventilatory requirement – ie increased demand for breathing at a given work rate – due to impaired gas transfer, eg as a result of ventilation/perfusion mismatching
▶ An increased central, cortical sensitization, often heightened by a vicious cycle of anxiety, exercise avoidance and deconditioning. This results in the inability to distinguish real 'physiological' breathlessness associated with lack of fitness from breathlessness directly related to the underlying condition

'high tech' facilities, provided that methods of testing are standardised. Recommendations for the use of these tests are available[2] and further statements on their local implementation will be forthcoming from the British Thoracic Society, who will shortly publish a consultative document, *Pulmonary Rehabilitation – Guidelines for Implementation.*

A fundamental part of the process is the identification of realistic objectives that the patient can expect to achieve by participation in an exercise programme. Published data have shown that the exercise tolerance of patients with COPD will improve in proportion to the total 'dose' of exercise (a combination of the intensity, duration and frequency of exercise sessions over a sustained period). Exercise training does not produce measurable improvements in the underlying respiratory impairment in patients with chronic respiratory disease, but rather reduces the disabling effects of the illness on normal daily functioning. Realistic objectives are paramount.

Some patients with moderately severe COPD can participate in sufficiently intensive aerobic exercise programmes (eg 80% of peak work rate) to improve peak work rate, endurance at a submaximal work rate, kinetics of oxygen uptake, CO_2 output, ventilation and heart rate, dead space : tidal volume ratio and total ventilation.[8] The programmes which are offered usually use walking and cycling, singly or in combination, in supervised training sessions of at least 20 minutes duration, 2–5 times per week for 4–12 weeks.

Patients who would be unable to participate in such programmes at the exercise intensity required, because of limiting symptoms such as breathlessness, can still improve their general exercise tolerance using more flexible programmes which allow training at lower work rates.[2]

For patients with even more severe disease, the objective may be to improve mobility and general conditioning, with little likelihood of major improvement.

Exercise programme options

A simple method of programme organisation can be implemented.[9] Patients with COPD are first characterised as having mild, moderate or severe disease using broad bands of lung function abnormality (see Table 1). These categories are helpful in the initial selection process for specific programmes, with further refinement after assessment of the patient's capabilities during actual participation in exercise. Many district general hospitals routinely provide cardiopulmonary exercise testing as part of the next step in the evaluation of patients with heart and lung disease. This can be helpful to identify co-existing conditions such as ischaemic heart disease, and to determine the physiological demand on the respiratory system during exercise at relatively high work rates. The importance of such evaluation lies in the fact that patients with the same FEV_1 may have markedly differing levels of exercise tolerance. Some patients may also allow arterial oxygen desaturation to progress to extreme levels during exercise without sensing a requirement to stop.

Table 1. Characterisation of COPD.

Severity of disease	Percentage of normal predicted values of FEV_1
Mild	>60
Moderate	40–60
Severe	<40

FEV_1 = Forced expiratory volume in one second.

High intensity endurance training

For patients with mild disease, progression to high intensity endurance training may be a realistic option, using heart rate monitors to standardise exercise intensity, just as sometimes advised for previously sedentary but otherwise normal subjects.[10] Nevertheless, many patients with mild COPD have had a very sedentary lifestyle and require a period of familiarisation before participating in the full programme, if only to ensure they remain motivated. The standard modes of training such as running, cycling, stepmaster and rowing can be used interchangeably, according to local access and patient preference. Treadmill or stepmaster support bars can be helpful to patients with COPD as they facilitate fixation of the upper limb girdle, allowing the accessory muscles of respiration to support breathing during aerobic exercise.

Moderate intensity endurance training

In practice, many patients with chronic lung disease cannot maintain such high intensity of work for long enough to complete the session and an acceptable compromise is to train at a lower intensity, equivalent to 60–70% of the maximal work rate achievable in the initial exercise evaluation. This allows the training exercise to be maintained for the duration of session required. The modes of exercise commonly used are brisk walking, cycling or gymnasium activities at the intensity that the patient has been found empirically to tolerate. It is important to note that patients with chronic lung disease should be supervised, preferably for at least two of the three training sessions required per week, to ensure that this subjective approach remains safe and effective. Currently, recommendations are that only 8 to10 patients can be supervised per session. An important aid to training is the patient's increasing awareness of how to interpret symptoms. A modification of the Borg scale for rating perceived exertion[11] is routinely used in exercise programmes for patients with chronic lung disease to describe levels of breathlessness. In practice, patients in formal pulmonary rehabilitation programmes usually use a combination of heart rate monitoring and perceived breathlessness to determine the work rate throughout an exercise session.

Strength training

An alternative to symptom-limited aerobic exercise programmes for patients with mild to moderate COPD is multi-gym weight training. Peripheral muscle weakness is reduced by this direct approach and endurance during treadmill walking also improves.[12] Training is based on repetitive contractions against 60–80% of the one-repetition maximum (ie 60–80% of the maximal weight lifted by the patient in a single contraction during preliminary exercise testing). Three sets of repetitions of each exercise are performed, with a rest between sets. Two sessions per week are the minimum required. The provision of small mobile weights is desirable as it allows a third session at home. At each session, the patient completes a circuit of exercises, systematically engaging upper and lower limbs, according to their individual prescription. While the order of exercises is not critical, they must be preceded by five-minute periods of stretching exercises designed to prevent muscle, tendon and ligament injuries. This type of training does not require monitoring of heart rate, as the objective is not cardiovascular conditioning. However, in practice, these exercises can make the patient breathless, and thus the Borg scale for breathlessness can be used to allow self assessment and to determine adequate recovery times between exercises.

Low intensity training

For patients with moderate to severe disease, who are unable to participate in the programmes already described, increased movement is the objective. These patients often have difficulty with the most basic of daily tasks such as walking, dressing, washing and housework. Therefore, the mobility programme should be designed gently to restore locomotive function of individual joints, muscles, ligaments and tendons by a series of careful stretching exercises plus gentle repetitions of muscle contraction and relaxation. By exercising each muscle group sequentially in isolation and unloaded, breathlessness is minimised, as is the risk of musculoskeletal injury. Examples of programmes used are given elsewhere[9] and include simple adaptations of routine gymnasium exercises such as 'wall' press-ups performed standing, and seated stomach muscle exercises, both designed to avoid undue breathlessness produced by lying flat. The main attractions of such a programme are that it can be performed by the most severely disabled patient and that it can be performed at home once the patient has learned the techniques under careful supervision. These patients are, in effect, doing circuit training of the individual muscle groups, and breathlessness is rarely such as to prevent completion. These programmes are of use, not only for patients at the severe end of the spectrum of disease, but also as an introductory programme for patients who have had many years of major inactivity, as a prelude to the next step of more intensive exercises. Furthermore, the mobility programme is a very important way of keeping patients involved in exercise during recovery from the inevitable acute exacerbations of their illness. Demotivation is, otherwise, very common, resulting from a perceived 'failure' to complete the full programme. Such patients need the companionship and sense of momentum that participation in the mobility programme can offer without any adverse effect.

Continuing care after completion of hospital-based programmes

There is an increasing interest in the provision of ongoing pulmonary rehabilitation programmes in primary care. The Department of Respiratory Medicine at Hairmyres Hospital has developed a collaborative scheme with the local authority South Lanarkshire Council; on completion of a 12-week hospital-based programme, patients transfer to local community sport and leisure centres. Several issues are critical to the success of this approach. The first is that the fitness trainers on site in the leisure centres undergo a training programme identifying the basic problems and needs of patients with chronic lung disease, with particular emphasis on exercise limitation. Secondly, patients are given concessionary rates to join the leisure centre and undergo an induction at the leisure centre under the combined supervision of the hospital physiotherapist and the centre's fitness trainer (who has received details of the individual patient's treatment plan and the problems they have encountered in the previous months). This liaison is critical, and is proving highly successful in allaying the fears of leisure centre staff in dealing with this particular client group. Thirdly, responsibility is clearly designated as remaining with the patient and not the leisure centre.

To date, this programme is highly successful, largely because the patients are themselves experienced in exercise participation. Patients who have reached this stage have already shown a commitment and consistency in approach that is likely to ensure successful, continuing self management. They are encouraged to view themselves as programme 'graduates' who leave the protected short-term process within hospital facilities to translate the improvements into routine daily living. Initial observations of the pilot collaborative study indicate very high satisfaction rates and ongoing commitment. (Further information regarding this pilot project can be obtained from the author and/or direct from the Administration Office, Blantyre Sports Centre, Blantyre, Lanarkshire).

Special considerations

Patients requiring oxygen therapy

During the period of evaluation at the hospital the presence or absence of exercise-induced oxygen desaturation will have been assessed. Some patients will require supplementary oxygen in order to maintain an arterial oxygen saturation >90% during exercise. It is not known whether this improves the efficacy of their training but it is of medicolegal importance, to reduce the theoretical possibility of adverse effects resulting from the stress of hypoxic exercise. In the UK, patients do not have routine access to portable oxygen by NHS prescription. Instead, supplementary oxygen for home exercise may be delivered from a renewable oxygen cylinder provided by arrangement with the GP and local pharmacist. Alternatively, for those who are eligible for long-term domiciliary oxygen (ie those with an arterial PO_2 <7.3kPa at rest), supplementary oxygen for low intensity home exercise may be delivered from an oxygen concentrator.

Steroid induced osteoporosis

Patients who have been taking long-term oral steroid therapy are likely to have osteoporosis. This is not a contra-indication to exercise but needs to be carefully considered by the physiotherapist in terms of the specific exercises offered. These may require modification, for example, in order to avoid spinal loading in flexion.

References

1 Lacasse Y, Wong E, Guyatt GH, *et al*. Meta-analysis of respiratory rehabilitation in chronic obstructive pulmonary disease. *Lancet* 1996; **348**: 1115–9.

2 American Thoracic Society. Pulmonary rehabilitation – 1999. *Am J Respir Crit Care Med* 1999; **159**: 1666–82.

3 American College of Chest Physicians and American Association of Cardiovascular and Pulmonary Rehabilitation. Pulmonary rehabilitation: joint ACCP-AACVPR evidence-based guidelines. *Chest* 1997; **112**: 1363–96.

4 Hamilton AL, Killian KJ, Summers E, Jones NL. Symptom intensity and subjective limitation to exercise in patients with cardiorespiratory disorders. *Chest* 1996; **110**: 1255–63.

5 Hamilton AL, Killian KJ, Summers E, Jones NL. Muscle strength, symptom intensity, and exercise capacity in patients with cardiorespiratory disorders. *Am J Respir Crit Care Med* 1995; **152**: 2021–31.

6 Butland RJA, Pang J, Gross ER, *et al*. Two-, six-, and 12-minute walking tests in respiratory disease. *Brit Med J* 1982; **284**: 1607–8.

7 Singh SJ, Morgan MDL, Scott S, *et al*. Development of a shuttle walking test of disability in patients with chronic airways obstruction. *Thorax* 1992; **47**: 1019–24.

8 Casaburi R, Patessio A, Ioli F, *et al*. Reductions in exercise lactic acidosis and ventilation as a result of exercise training in patients with obstructive lung disease. *Am Rev Respir Dis* 1991; **143**: 9–18.

9 Clark CJ. Pulmonary rehabilitation in chronic respiratory insufficiency. Setting up a pulmonary rehabilitation programme. *Thorax* 1994; **49**: 270–8.

10 American College of Sports Medicine. *ACSM's Guidelines for Graded Exercise Testing and Exercise Prescription (6 ed)*. Philadelphia: Lippincott, Williams & Wilkins, 2000.

11 Burdon JGW, Juniper EF, Killian KJ, *et al*. The perception of breathlessness in asthma. *Am Rev Respir Dis* 1982; **126**: 825–8.

12 Clark CJ, Cochrane LM, Mackay E, Paton B. Skeletal muscle strength and endurance in patients with mild COPD and the effects of weight training. *Eur Respir J* 2000; **15**: 92–7. [Erratum in *Eur Respir J* 2000; **15**: 816.]

10 | Delivering an exercise prescription for a healthier childhood

Neil Armstrong

Introduction

Regular physical activity and higher aerobic fitness lower overall adult mortality in a dose-response manner and the beneficial effects of appropriate physical activity during adult life are extensively documented.[1] The benefits of physical activity during childhood and adolescence have been studied less frequently but appropriate physical activity during youth has been demonstrated to increase aspects of health and well-being (Box 1).[2-4] However, recommending an exercise prescription that is based on sound experimental evidence and is appropriate for all children and adolescents is not currently possible. A consensus exists concerning the types of exercise most likely to promote aspects of health and well-being during youth but dose-response data are not available.

Physical activity and aerobic fitness

Few studies have reported the responses of children and adolescents to well-designed and rigorously controlled exercise training programmes.

Box 1
Benefits of physical activity and exercise training during youth:

▶ Increases aerobic fitness
▶ Increases muscle strength
▶ Improves flexibility
▶ Reduces body fatness
▶ Aids management of obesity
▶ Lowers high blood pressure
▶ Promotes skeletal health
▶ Enhances psychological well-being
▶ Raises quality of life

Studies with girls are particularly sparse. The optimal exercise prescription for young people is yet to be designed and reliable dose-response data are non-existent. Nevertheless, there is general agreement that the type of exercise most likely to increase aerobic fitness, as defined by peak $\dot{V}O_2$, is rhythmical movement of large muscle groups for sustained periods of time (eg running, cycling, swimming). Box 2 outlines an exercise prescription which, if adhered to for 12 weeks or longer, would be expected to induce significant increases in the aerobic fitness of both boys and girls. The magnitude of the increases, however, may be less than those expected with adult subjects and some studies, particularly those with prepubertal children, have reported no changes in aerobic fitness following a training programme but the hypothesis that there is a critical period of enhanced responses to exercise training remains to be proven. Exercise training during childhood and adolescence does not induce permanent increases in aerobic fitness and once training stops its effects decay.[2,5,6]

Box 2
Exercise prescription for the improvement of aerobic fitness
(Adapted from ref [2])

▶ Frequency   3–5 times per week
▶ Intensity   80–90% of maximal heart rate
                      (ie 160 to 180 bpm)
▶ Duration   20–30 minutes at above intensity
▶ Type   Rhythmic exercise using large muscle groups, eg running, cycling, swimming

---

Physical activity and muscle strength

Adolescents respond to resistance training programmes with muscle hypertrophy and increased muscle strength, although girls may experience a less dramatic response than boys. There is a popular view that resistance training programmes are ineffective with prepubescent children. This is not based on sound scientific evidence, and well-controlled studies have clearly demonstrated that appropriate resistance training programmes can increase muscle strength during childhood. Prepubescent children do not normally experience significant increases in muscle size with resistance training, and observed increases in strength are primarily due to neurological adaptation. Significant increases in motor unit activation have been noted following resistance training and this, coupled with improvements in motor co-ordination, is the likely explanation for prepubescent strength increases in the absence of muscle hypertrophy.[2,6,7]

If resistance training programmes are closely supervised and consistent with the recommendation that children and adolescents should avoid the repetitive use of maximal resistance,[8] they are no more likely to cause musculoskeletal injury than participation in many popular sports.[9] Box 3 describes an appropriate resistance training prescription for young people.

Training-induced strength gains will not persist through a period of detraining, and once training ceases its effects decay. The long-term benefits of resistance training depend upon the maintenance of the programme into adult life.

Box 3
A progressive overload resistance training programme

- ▶ Frequency   2–3 times per week
- ▶ Intensity   8–12 RM* per set for upper limb exercises
                        15–20 RM* per set for lower limb exercises
- ▶ Duration   1–3 sets of exercise for each muscle group to be trained
- ▶ Type   Weight training

*A repetition maximum (RM) is the maximal load that a muscle group can lift over a given number of repetitions before fatiguing. For upper limb exercise the 8 RM load is determined and the programme implemented. As training progresses the overload is increased by the number of repetitions until 12 is achieved. The new 8 RM is then determined and the process repeated over time. (Adapted from ref [2] and based on recommendations from Sale[10] and Kraemer, et al [11]).

Physical activity and flexibility

Stretching exercises to improve flexibility can be either ballistic or static. Ballistic stretching uses momentum to produce the stretch by 'bouncing' within a stretched position. As this type of stretching is associated with a high risk of injury it is not recommended. Static stretching exercises involve stretching a muscle comfortably beyond its normal length and holding the stretch. They can significantly improve flexibility with little risk of muscle tears and soreness and are therefore the preferred method for flexibility training (see Box 4). Assisted passive stretching and the use of proprioceptive neuromuscular facilitation are advanced stretching techniques which have been shown to be successful in increasing flexibility, however, to avoid injury young people should use them cautiously.[12–14]

Box 4
Exercise prescription guidelines for improving flexibility. (Adapted from ref [2])

▶ Frequency   3–7 times per week
▶ Intensity   Muscle should be stretched beyond its normal length
▶ Duration   The stretch should be held for about 6–10 sec and repeated three times, without bouncing
▶ Type   Static stretching

Physical activity and body fatness

There is a minor to moderate relationship between habitual physical activity and body fatness and, on balance, obese young people tend to be less physically active than their leaner peers. However, obese or overweight youngsters may well expend more energy than those of normal body mass despite being physically less active. Aerobic fitness is not necessarily impaired in obese or overweight young people but they are disadvantaged in activities which require their body mass to be supported.

Aerobic exercise training (Box 2) induces small reductions in adiposity in both obese and non-obese young people. More significant changes in body composition occur if the exercise programme is supplemented with a concurrent dietary modification programme. Physical activity also has positive effects on blood lipid profile, blood pressure and glucose metabolism in obese young people despite only minor changes in body fatness. However, despite the positive effects of aerobic exercise training programmes, follow-up studies have indicated high recidivism. Prescriptions to promote lifestyle modification and increase energy expenditure are essential to long-term success in management of obesity (Box 5).[2,15,16]

Physical activity and blood pressure

In studies where body fatness has been appropriately controlled for, relationships between habitual physical activity (or aerobic fitness) and blood pressure have seldom reached statistical significance. Similarly, there is little consistent evidence to support the efficacy of exercise training in reducing resting blood pressure in normotensive young

Box 5
Physical activity programme for the management of obesity during youth (Adapted from ref [2] and based on recommendations from Bar-Or[15])

► Emphasize the use of large muscle groups
► Move the whole body over distance
► Emphasize duration rather than intensity of exercise
► Raise daily energy expenditure by 10–15%
► Include activities to promote muscle strength
► Include daily (habitual) physical activities
► Increase the volume of physical activity progressively
► Incorporate the young person's preferred activities

people. Several studies, however, have demonstrated significant reductions in both diastolic (DBP) and systolic (SBP) blood pressure in hypertensive young people.[2,17] Hagberg and his colleagues[18,19] have provided the most valuable insights into the effects of exercise training on hypertensive adolescents. They investigated the effects of six months endurance running (Box 6) on 25 adolescents whose blood pressure was persistently above the 95th percentile for their age and sex. Both DBP and SBP decreased significantly although no significant change in either body mass or fatness was detected. When the subjects were re-assessed nine months after the cessation of the training programme, SBP had returned to pre-training levels but DBP was still significantly below pre-training levels in the subjects who initially had diastolic hypertension. Five of the subjects continued with a five month resistance training programme immediately following the endurance training programme. The SBP of the weight training group remained significantly lower than when measured at the beginning of the project. The two subjects who

Box 6
Exercise training programme to reduce the blood pressure of young people with hypertension (From Hagberg, et al[18,19])

► Frequency   3 times per week
► Intensity   60–65% of peak $\dot{V}O_2$
► Duration   40 minutes
► Type   Running

initially had diastolic hypertension maintained the reduction in DBP achieved by endurance training.

Physical activity and skeletal health

Increasing bone mineral density (BMD) during childhood and adolescence may reduce the risk of osteoporosis in adult life. Although much of the variability in BMD may be attributed to hormonal status and to genetics, peak BMD is also dependent upon environmental factors, particularly nutrition and physical activity.

Adequate nutrition is vital during growth and maturation and sufficient calcium in the diet appears to be a prerequisite for skeletal health. The positive effects of calcium intake and physical activity on skeletal health may be independent but it is possible that calcium is an important enabling factor for the effects of physical activity on BMD.

Well controlled, prospective studies of the effect of physical activity on BMD are sparse and the results are equivocal. However, active young people have higher BMD than their less active peers and comparisons of trained and untrained subjects have provided evidence of a positive association between participation in weightbearing sports and BMD.

The mode of exercise that best promotes BMD is yet to be determined but skeletal loading studies in animals suggest that physical activity, designed to increase BMD and bone strength, should involve loads of high magnitude and high rate, should be intermittent in nature, and should involve varied and diverse patterns of stress. Activities such as walking and jogging have been recommended for the promotion of skeletal health but peak strain magnitudes during this type of physical activity are not particularly high and strain distribution is not altered to a great degree. Weight (resistance) training offers skeletal loading of high magnitude and varied patterns of stress through lifting exercises with strain distributions which are different from those encountered in normal daily activities. In weight lifting, however, loading is more static in nature and is applied at lower rates than in activities such as running.

De-training studies with children and adolescents are not available. However, in adults BMD regresses towards its pre-training value following a period of de-training. Similarly, in both adults and children periods of immobilization are detrimental to skeletal health.

Current data do not allow an evidence-based exercise prescription for the promotion of skeletal health but expert opinion suggests that an appropriate prescription would promote lifetime participation in weightbearing physical activities supplemented by resistance training.[2,20,21]

Physical activity, psychological health and well-being

Physical activity improves self-esteem and reduces anxiety, stress and depression. The mechanisms by which it may influence young people's psychological well-being are not well understood and its value as a treatment for clinically diagnosed mental health problems remains to be established.[22–24]

The specific effects of various types of physical activity on mental health have not been documented and there are no dose-response data from well-controlled studies. Calfas and Taylor[22] reviewed the extant literature and recommended an exercise prescription similar to that described in Box 2 but with a reduced intensity of 70% of maximal heart rate. A more appropriate behavioural goal may be for children and adolescents to adopt active lifestyles. As enjoyable early activity experiences are more likely to foster future participation perhaps young people should be encouraged to develop a repertoire of motor skills, so that they may achieve success in a range of activities and feel confident enough in their own abilities to want to pursue more active lifestyles.

Physical activity

Although there are direct health benefits from appropriate physical activity during childhood and adolescence more research is required to establish dose-response data suitable for the recommendation of specific exercise prescriptions. Recent emphasis has therefore been on the establishment of recommendations for young people's daily volume of physical activity. Three major consensus conferences have reviewed the existing data, taken expert opinion, and produced authoritative guidelines (Box 7).[4,25,26]

In 1993, an International Consensus Conference on Physical Activity Guidelines for Adolescents produced two recommendations.[25] The first focused on increasing daily physical activity in the context of family, school and community activities. The second emphasised the importance of sustained ($\geq$20 min) physical activities requiring moderate to vigorous levels of exertion, where moderate activity was defined as equivalent to brisk walking and vigorous activity was related to activities such as jogging (Box 7). Subsequent conferences[4,26] have moved away from the requirement of sustained moderate to vigorous physical activity and recommended the daily accumulation of moderate physical activity (Box 7).

The assessment of children's physical activity is one of the most difficult tasks in epidemiological research.[5,27,28] A recent review[5] of the literature located only 13 studies which have monitored young people's physical activity over at least three full days, and only seven of the studies had even moderate sample sizes.

Nevertheless, data have been generally consistent and can be illustrated using a series of studies in which the heart rates of 839 young people, aged 5–16 years, from South-West England were monitored continuously for at least three weekdays.[29] To interpret the heart rate data, ninety-eight 5–16-year-olds were exercised at various speeds on a horizontal treadmill and it was noted that, regardless of age, brisk walking and jogging elicited steady-state heart rates of about 140 and 160 bpm respectively.

Twenty minute periods of either moderate (heart rate ≥140 bpm) or vigorous (heart rate ≥160 bpm) physical activity were rare in all age groups. Eighty four percent of girls and 77% of boys did not experience a

---

Box 7
Physical activity recommendations for young people:

Sallis & Patrick[25]

▶ All adolescents should be physically active daily, or nearly every day, as part of play, games, sports, work, transportation, recreation, physical education, or planned exercise, in the context of family, school and community activities

▶ Adolescents should engage in three or more sessions per week of activities that each last ≥20 min and that require moderate to vigorous levels of exertion

Health Education Authority[4]

▶ All young people should participate in physical activity of at least moderate intensity for one hour per day

▶ Young people who currently do little activity should participate in physical activity of at least moderate intensity for at least 30 min per day

▶ At least twice a week, some of these activities should help to enhance and maintain muscular strength and flexibility, and bone health

National Institutes of Health[26]

▶ All children and adults should set and reach a goal of accumulating at least 30 min of moderate-intensity physical activity on most, and preferably all, days of the week. Those who currently meet these standards may derive additional health and fitness benefits by becoming more physically active or including more vigorous activity.

single 20 min period of vigorous activity in three days of monitoring. All the girls and over 97% of the boys did not experience the equivalent of a daily 20 min period of vigorous activity.

Fifty percent of 10–16 year-old girls and 38% of similarly aged boys did not even experience a 10 min period of moderate physical activity. Ten minute periods equivalent to moderate activity were more common amongst young children, but 31% of girls and 14% of boys did not raise their heart rate ≥140 bpm for a sustained 10 min period.

When the data were re-analysed to address the recommendation of accumulating daily 30 min of moderate physical activity, it was shown that the vast majority of young children (6–10 years) accumulate a daily total of at least 30 min with the heart rate ≥140 bpm, although more boys than girls do so. However, there is a steady decline with age in the percentage of young people who achieve this target, with boys outscoring girls at all ages (Fig 1 and Box 8).

Promoting physical activity

Some children and adolescents are physically active, but many young people have adopted sedentary lifestyles. Data to determine the trend of young people's physical activity over time are not available but an analysis of energy intake, data collected since 1930, indicate that there has been a

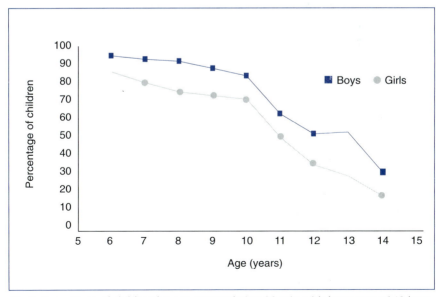

Fig 1. Percentage of children by age accumulating 30 min with heart rate ≥140 bpm. (Reproduced from ref [29] with permission)

Box 8
Young people's physical activity patterns:

▶ Sustained periods of moderate to vigorous physical activity are seldom experienced by many youngsters.

▶ Girls are less likely to experience sustained periods of moderate to vigorous physical activity than boys.

▶ Daily accumulation of moderate physical activity is higher in boys than girls from an early age but it decreases with age in both sexes.

---

marked reduction in energy intake without a reduction in body mass.[30] This must reflect a diminished energy expenditure and suggests that children and adolescents have become more sedentary over the past 60 years. An appropriate strategy for health promotion is therefore to foster active lifestyles.

No prospective study has followed children into middle age and beyond but physical activity appears to track at weak to moderate levels during adolescence, from adolescence into adulthood and across various ages during adult life.[31] Data do support the premise that inactive young people are unlikely to become active adults.[32] So, as adult physical activity patterns may be established during youth, strategies for physical activity promotion should have a lifetime dimension.

The myriad of interacting factors which may influence young people's physical activity are not understood fully but the consensus view is that no single correlate explains physical activity behaviour. Wide ranging discussion encompassing, for example, the role of government departments, local authorities, the community, the media, the family, the 'active' school, the physical education programme and peer pressure are readily available elsewhere.[2-4,33] This paper focuses on the potential impact of doctors on physical activity promotion.

Doctors and other healthcare professionals[8,34-7] have a high credibility among children and adolescents, which may be influential in promoting young people's daily physical activity; but data are sparse. In the *American Medical Association Guidelines for Adolescent Preventive Health Services* at least two recommendations specifically target the role of the doctor in promoting youth physical activity (Box 9).[38]

Several effective programmes promoting behaviours such as physical activity have used a social cognitive approach.[39] Social cognitive theory suggests that self-efficacy (confidence in one's ability to perform a task) is

> **Box 9**
> **American Medical Association guidelines for adolescent preventive health services (From Elster and Kuznets[38])**
>
> ▶ All adolescents should receive health guidance annually to promote the reduction of injuries. Health guidance for injury prevention includes counselling to promote appropriate physical conditioning before exercise. (Recommendation 6)
> ▶ All adolescents should receive health guidance annually about the benefits of exercise and should be encouraged to engage in safe exercise on regular basis. (Recommendation 8)

the primary psychological determinant of behaviour but also acknowledges the influence of social factors and role models. The theory has been reviewed elsewhere in the context of youth physical activity promotion[33] and with specific reference to the role of health care providers in promoting youth physical activities.[37] DuRant and Hergenroeder[37] apply social cognitive theory and adapt the GAPS model (Box 10) to address the promotion of youth physical activity in the American doctor's office or clinic and the following section is drawn from their paper.

Gather information

The doctor should initially determine if the young person is sedentary (see Box 7) and assess his/her beliefs and attitudes to physical activity. An annual examination may be the most appropriate setting for an interview which should be interactive and non-judgemental.

> **Box 10**
> **The GAPS model (From DuRant and Hergenroeder[37])**
>
> G = Gather information
> A = Assess further
> P = Problem identification, pros and cons, plan
> S = Self-efficacy, solving barriers, shake on a contract

Assess further

If the youngster is physically active then the doctor should provide positive reinforcement and perhaps advise on appropriate stretching and warm-ups before exercise and other techniques to avoid injury during exercise. Information on the availability of local active leisure pursuits could be provided. If the young person is sedentary, then the doctor moves to the next stage of the intervention.

Problem identification, pros and cons, plan

In this phase, the youngster and the doctor need to agree that a problem exists and determine what behaviours the young person is willing to change. Specific goals can be set and a plan for a change in physical activity habits developed. Potential barriers to engaging in physical activity need to be identified in relation to the young person's physiological, psychological and social development. Implicit in this phase is the doctor's ability to offer appropriate exercise prescriptions.

Self-efficacy

Once goals have been set and an initial plan has been developed perceived barriers and possible solutions need to be discussed further. Family and peer support may be necessary to initiate and sustain the agreed activity programme. The doctor could help to devise a weekly schedule and provide easy-to-use physical activity diaries which can be completed and brought to the subsequent consultation. To build self-efficacy physical activity goals should be realistic, easily accomplishable and progressive. Positive reinforcement increases the likelihood that a behaviour change will be sustained. For example, health centre staff could make a follow-up call to ask the young person how the programme is progressing and offer further advice.

Doctors are, of course, not limited to promoting youth physical activity in their clinic and those with the expertise and interest can have a major impact on local health initiatives,[40] in the local community[2, 41] and in local schools.[2,42] The role of doctors in the prevention and rehabilitation of youth sports injuries is reviewed in detail elsewhere[3] as is the design of exercise prescriptions for children with chronic health conditions.[3,43]

References

1   US Department of Health and Human Services. *Physical Activity and Health: A Report of the Surgeon General.* Atlanta, GA: US Department of Health and

Human Services, Centres for Disease Control and Prevention, National Centre for Chronic Disease Prevention and Health Promotion, 1996.

2 Armstrong N, Welsman JR. *Young People and Physical Activity.* Oxford: Oxford University Press, 1997.

3 Armstrong N, VanMechelen W (eds). *Paediatric Exercise Science and Medicine.* Oxford: Oxford University Press, 2000.

4 Biddle S, Sallis J, Cavill N. *Young and Active?* London: Health Education Authority, 1998.

5 Armstrong N. Physical fitness and physical activity during childhood and adolescence. In: Chan KM, Micheli L (eds). *Sports and Children.* Hong Kong: Williams and Wilkins, 1998.

6 Mahon A. Exercise training. In: Armstrong N, Van Mechelen W (eds). *Paediatric Exercise Science and Medicine.* Oxford: Oxford University Press, 2000.

7 Blimkie CJR, Sale DG. Strength development and trainability during childhood. In: Van Praagh E (ed). *Pediatric Anaerobic Performance.* Champaign, Illinois: Human Kinetics, 1998.

8 American Academy of Pediatrics. Fitness in the pre-school child. *Pediatrics* 1976; **58**: 88–9.

9 Blimkie CJR. Benefits and risks of resistance training in children. In: Cahill BR, Pearl AJ (eds). *Intensive Participation in Children's Sports.* Champaign, Illinois: Human Kinetics, 1993.

10 Sale DG. Strength training in children. In: Gisolfi CV, Lamb DR (eds). *Perspectives in Exercise Science and Sports Medicine, vol 2 - Youth, Exercise and Sport.* Indianapolis: Benchmark Press, 1989.

11 Kraemer WJ, Fry AC, Frykman PN, *et al.* Resistance training and youth. *Pediatr Exerc Sci* 1989; **1**: 336–50.

12 Brodie DA, Royce J. Developing flexibility during childhood and adolescence. In: VanPraagh E (ed). *Pediatric Anaerobic Performance.* Champaign, Illinois: Human Kinetics, 1998.

13 McNaught-Davis P. *Flexibility.* London: Partridge Press, 1991.

14 Alter MJ. *Science of Stretching.* Champaign, Illinois: Human Kinetics, 1988.

15 Bar-Or O. Obesity. In: Goldberg B (ed). *Sports and Exercise for Children with Chronic Health Conditions.* Champaign, Illinois: Human Kinetics, 1995.

16 Bar-Or O, Baranowski T. Physical activity, adiposity, and obesity among adolescents. *Pediatr Exerc Sci* 1994; **6**: 348–60.

17 Alpert BS, Wilmore JH. Physical activity and blood pressure in adolescents. *Pediatr Exerc Sci* 1994; **6**: 361–80.

18 Hagberg JM, Goldring D, Eshami AA, *et al.* Effects of exercise training on the blood pressure and hemodymanics of adolescent hypertensives. *Am J Cardiol* 1983; **52**: 763–8.

19 Hagberg JM, Ehsani AA, Goldring D, *et al.* Effect of weight training on blood pressure and hemodynamics in hypertensive adolescents. *J Pediatr* 1984; **104**: 147–51.

20 Bailey DA, Martin AD. Physical activity and skeletal health in adolescents. *Pediatr Exerc Sci* 1994; **6**: 330–47.

21 Kemper HCG. Physical activity, physical fitness and bone health. In: Armstrong N, VanMechelen W (eds). *Paediatric Exercise Science and Medicine.* Oxford: Oxford University Press, 2000.

22 Calfas KJ, Taylor WC. Effects of physical activity on psychological variables in adolescents. *Pediatr Exerc Sci* 1994; **6**: 406–23.

23 Mutrie N, Parfitt G. Physical activity and its link with mental, social and moral health in young people. In: Biddle S, Sallis J, Cavill N (eds). *Young and Active?* London: HEA, 1998.

24 Tortolero SR, Taylor WC, Murray NG. Physical activity, physical fitness and social, psychological, and emotional health. In: Armstrong N, VanMechelen W (eds). *Paediatric Exercise Science and Medicine.* Oxford: Oxford University Press, 2000.

25 Sallis JF, Patrick K. Physical activity guidelines for adolescents: A consensus statement. *Pediatr Exerc Sci* 1994; **6**: 302–14.

26 National Institutes of Health Consensus Development Panel on Physical Activity and Cardiovascular Health. Physical activity and cardiovascular health. *JAMA* 1996; **276**: 241–6.

27 Armstrong N, VanMechelen W. How fit and active are children and youth? In: Biddle S, Cavill N, Sallis J (eds). *Young and Active?* London: HEA, 1998.

28 Harro M, Riddoch C. Physical activity. In: Armstrong N, Van Mechelen W (eds). *Paediatric Exercise Science and Medicine.* Oxford: Oxford University Press, 2000.

29 Armstrong N. Young people's physical activity patterns as assessed by heart rate monitoring. *J Sports Sci* 1998; **16**: S9–S16.

30 Durnin JVGA. Physical activity levels past and present. In: Norgan N (ed). *Physical Activity and Health.* Cambridge: University Press, 1992.

31 Malina RM. Tracking of physical activity and physical fitness across the lifespan. *Res Q Exerc Sport* 1996; **67**: 48–57.

32 Activity and Health Research. *Allied Dunbar national fitness survey.* London: Sports Council and Health Education Authority, 1992.

33 Sallis JF. Determinants of physical activity behaviour in children. In: Pate RR, Hohn RC (eds). *Health and Fitness through Physical Education.* Champaign, Illinois: Human Kinetics, 1994.

34 American College of Sports Medicine. Opinion statement on physical fitness in children and youth. *Med Sci Sports Exerc* 1988; **20**: 422–3.

35 Strong WB. Physical activity and children. *Circulation* 1990; **81**: 1697–701.

36 Armstrong N. Promoting physical activity in schools. *Health Visitor* 1993; **66**: 362–4.

37 DuRant RH, Hergenroeder AC. Promotion of physical activity among adolescents by primary health care providers. *Pediatr Exerc Sci* 1994; **6**: 448–63.

38 Elster AB, Kuznets NJ. *American Medical Association's Guidelines for Adolescent Preventive Health Services.* Baltimore: Williams and Wilkins, 1994.

39 Bandura A. *Social Foundations of Thought and Action.* Englewood Cliffs, New Jersey: Prentice-Hall, 1986.

40 Health Education Authority. *Young People and Physical Activity. Promoting Better Practices.* London: Health Education Authority, 1997.

41 Salis J. Family and community interventions to promote physical activity in young people. In: Biddle S, Sallis J, Cavill N (eds). *Young and Active?* London: Health Education Authority, 1998.

42 Health Education. Health promoting schools. *Health Ed* 2000; **100**: 102–30.

43 Goldberg B. *Sports and Exercise for Children with Chronic Health Conditions.* Champaign, Illinois: Human Kinetics, 1995.

11 | Delivering an exercise prescription for patients with disabilities

Nick Webborn

Introduction

The importance of maintaining physical activity for longevity is now firmly established in the scientific literature.[1,2] It is important in the prevention and management of many of the major diseases encountered in modern medical practice.[3,4] Indeed, one of the major challenges for the next millennium will be to persuade the general population of its importance, and to persuade them to move away from their sedentary lifestyles. These potential benefits are also available to people with physical disabilities but they will require specific advice and assistance from the medical profession.

Encouraging physical activity for people with physical disabilities has been used for more than half a century in the rehabilitative process, but has only in more recent years been recognised as important for health maintenance. Sir Ludwig Guttman, at the Spinal Injuries Unit at Stoke Mandeville Hospital, introduced sport as part of the rehabilitation programme in the 1940s. Guttman believed that 'by restoring activity of mind and body – by instilling self-respect, self-discipline, a competitive spirit and comradeship – sport develops mental attitude through essential social reintegration'. He would have been surprised by the achievements of current paralympic athletes. A time of 1.5 hours for a paraplegic in a wheelchair marathon or a high jump of two metres by a single leg amputee, show that people with disabilities are capable of considerable athletic performance, given appropriate exercise training. It is important that these achievements are recognised by the medical profession to help alter attitudes to physical activity for people with disabilities, where many doctors are restrictive rather than prescriptive. While sport is not the focus of this article, the sporting achievements do show the potential elite levels of performance. The development of equipment and facilities that are disability specific has also widened the scope for people to participate in physical activity.

The problems of an ageing disabled population

There is a significant public health problem facing the nation as the result of an increasing ageing disabled population. As medical health care and technology moves on, so the number of people living with a disability increases. The management of the complications of, for example, spinal cord injury has improved such that the longevity of these patients has increased, leading to exposure to the diseases that result from a sedentary lifestyle. The current recommendation for physical activity for the general population is the accumulation of a minimum of 30 minutes of moderate intensity activity on at least five days per week.[5] The challenge for people with disabilities is to find safe and beneficial physical activities that are appropriate to their disability.

Barriers to physical activity for people with disabilities

Historically, there are several reasons why people with disabilities have less often had an active lifestyle. Parental over-protection[6] of a child with a disability is understandable. Nevertheless, it is important that parents are aware of the potential downside of a sedentary lifestyle and understand the potential benefits of improved self-esteem and self-efficacy by integration and inclusion within a physical activity programme.[7] Part of the problem, however, has been medical over-protection. It is well known that medical undergraduate and postgraduate programmes have neglected the benefits of physical activity. This applies even more when dealing with people with disabilities, and the view that 'perhaps it's safer not to' has been born out of ignorance. It is important to revise our medical education programmes in the light of current knowledge of the hazards of a sedentary lifestyle.

For many people their first introduction to organised physical activity is in childhood through the school system. In addition to a general reduction in physical activity during the school week, there is a reluctance to integrate children with disabilities into able-bodied sport in schools. There is also a general lack of organised sport programmes specifically for people with disabilities. The shortage of appropriate and accessible sporting facilities and the lack of coaches with appropriate knowledge and training also hamper those people with disabilities who do have an inclination towards increased physical activity.

Conditioning and monitoring

There are many desirable outcomes from increased physical activity. These include increased cardiovascular fitness, muscle strength, bone density and range of motion and flexibility in joints, as well as psychological and social benefits. This list is not exhaustive but when considering giving advice, one needs to take into account the potential for gain in each of these areas with regard to the individual's disability. For optimal health, all these components are desirable but possibly in different proportions. For example, for someone with paraplegia, regular workouts in a wheelchair or swimming will have beneficial effects on the cardiovascular system and increase muscle strength in the upper limbs. However, the absence of weight bearing activity will limit maintenance of bone density, and so the use of a standing frame may still be appropriate to stimulate osteoblastic activity while not being seen *per se* as physical activity.

To monitor training intensity, various adaptations may need to be made. For example, the energy cost of ambulation in cerebral palsy may be up to three times normal and therefore this needs to be considered when setting walking speed. The potential influence of certain medications on heart rate will need to be considered, particularly since medication use is more common in this group than in the average population. For those with a high spinal cord lesion at the level of T1 or above, adaptations will need to be made in setting heart rate responses. The absence of sympathetic cardiac innervation produces a depressed maximal heart rate. Maximal heart rates of between 110–130 bpm have been observed and are determined by intrinsic sino-atrial activity.[8] This reduction in heart rate reserve means that standard guidelines for heart rate responses to activity and threshold levels cannot be observed. The use of ratings of perceived exertion, however, appears to be as appropriate for wheelchair users as for ambulant users.[9]

Cautions

Provided the general principles of a gradual and progressive increase in training are followed, an improvement in cardiovascular fitness can be made in a variety of disabilities.[10] There are relatively few absolute contraindications to participation, but it is not only motor limitations which must be considered when advising someone with a disability about modes of physical activity. Certain diseases and syndromes will be associated with an increased incidence of cardiac disease and this may require evaluation if strenuous participation is intended. However, doctors should be cautious about excluding children from appropriate levels of activity on the basis of possible cardiac disease without good evidence.[11]

Some activities will have an increased risk for injury through collision, falling or physical contact. This is important for those with conditions where there is a reduction in bone mineral density secondary to immobilisation or as a primary cause (eg osteogenesis imperfecta). Subcutaneous pacemakers or CSF shunts may also be susceptible to trauma. It remains a subject of debate as to whether children with Down's Syndrome should undergo screening for atlanto-axial instability before taking part in some activities.[12]

People with disabilities taking part in regular physical activity are no less susceptible to overuse injuries than their able-bodied counterparts. Indeed, the risk factors are the same and they may be more prevalent in the group with disabilities. Biomechanical factors predispose towards certain injuries and different disabilities will provide different biomechanical challenges. Technical factors of sport are contributory sources of injury and it may not be possible for someone with a disability to achieve 'perfect technique' for a variety of reasons, including co-ordination difficulties, poor flexibility or muscle contractures.

Environmental issues are also important as the ability to generate or lose heat is affected in those with certain disabilities. For those with a spinal cord injury there will be reduction in the function of both the peripheral receptor and the heat loss mechanism below the level of the lesion. Paraplegics and tetraplegics exercising in a hot environment will be more susceptible to heat-related illness.[13] Not only do they have a basal sweat rate below the level of the spinal lesion; above this level, the sweat rates may be so high that the sweat may drip off instead of allowing evaporation and cooling to take place. Conversely, susceptibility to rapid cooling in cold environments and the possibility of circulatory disorders associated with the underlying condition may need appropriate clothing and headgear.

Choosing the activity or sport

Clearly, many medical issues must be addressed when advising someone with a disability about appropriate activities. For physical activity to be a long-term lifestyle, however, enjoyment is a crucial factor and the personal preference of the individual is important. Cognitive ability and the social skills of the person will also influence their ability to follow rules of games and the ability to interact socially with others. This may help influence whether an individual activity, group activity or team sport may be most appropriate.

Within the locality one will need to become aware of the facilities that can be provided in the community. The availability of appropriate and experienced coaching and support staff will also be a key determinant. A successful swim club for people with disabilities draws in other members of the local community to participate. Without this support it is less likely for people with disabilities voluntarily to participate in local swimming programmes. Contact with the local or regional sports development officer may help to locate existing groups currently functioning in the area. The English Federation for Disability Sport or similar organisations in Scotland, Wales and Northern Ireland are also sources of information.

The development of a variety of different sports for people with disabilities, particularly in the competitive environment has led to an increase in the technical complexity and expense of equipment. Wheelchairs adapted for different sports (eg tennis, rugby, basketball or road racing) are all different in design and usually cost more than £1,000. Although these sports specific chairs are not essential for participation at a basic level, once someone with a disability participates regularly in any of these sports, the cost of equipment may be a limiting factor.

As a general rule, activities and sports can be classified by their aerobic intensity, potential for trauma and demands for co-ordination. The various risks and potential benefits specific to the individual, their disability and their condition can then be matched with personal preference and local resources, in order to help the individual find a sustainable form of physical activity for long-term health. People with disabilities have taken part in virtually every sport available including high risk sports such as mountain climbing and sub aqua diving.

Historically, competitive sports for people with disabilities have developed within certain groups of people with broadly similar types of disability. These are usually divided into the following groups:

■ Spinal cord lesions, congenital or acquired

■ Visual impairment

■ Cerebral palsy

■ Amputees

■ 'Les Autres' – this is a term used for people with certain disabilities who do not fit into the traditional categories and include conditions such as muscular dystrophy or multiple sclerosis.

Each of the groups presents different challenges and these are beyond the scope of this article (see further reading).

Beneficial health outcomes

There is accumulating evidence that physically active disabled people make fewer visits to physicians and tend to have fewer medical complications and hospitalisations than their sedentary counterparts.[14] Paraplegic athletes were more successful than non-athletes in avoiding major medical complications of spinal cord injury.[15] Cooper and colleagues published a consensus statement regarding research on physical activity and health among people with disabilities in 1999.[16] They stated that as people with disabilities live longer, the need to address long-term health issues and risk of secondary disability must receive greater attention. They pointed towards five areas that required future work. These included:

▮ Epidemiological studies

▮ Effects of nutrition on health and the ability to exercise

▮ Cardiovascular and pulmonary health

▮ Children with disabilities

▮ Accessibility and safety of exercise programmes.

In summary, it is important that physicians and other health care workers recognise the potential health benefits from an increase in physical activity by people with disabilities. This needs to be promoted through primary and secondary health care providers but at the present time these people have inadequate knowledge to deliver the message appropriately. Improvement in undergraduate and postgraduate training with regard to exercise and health is important and needs to be addressed. Only then will it be possible for health workers to deliver the appropriate message to patients and parents. Within the community we need to support people with disabilities by providing appropriate facilities and equipment. In this way many physical, psychological and social benefits will be achieved which may have a significant impact on the cost of health care provision and quality of life.

References

1   Blair SN, Kohl HW 3rd, Barlow CE, *et al.* Changes in physical fitness and all-cause mortality. A prospective study of healthy and unhealthy men. *JAMA* 1995; **273**: 1093–8.

2   Wei M, Kampert JB, Barlow CE, *et al.* Relationship between low cardiorespiratory fitness and mortality in normal-weight, overweight, and obese men. *JAMA* 1999; **282**: 1547–53.

3   Kriska AM, Blair SN, Pereira MA. The potential role of physical activity in the prevention of non- insulin-dependent diabetes mellitus: the epidemiological evidence. *Exerc Sport Sci Rev* 1994; **22**: 121–43.

4   Smith SC, Jr., Blair SN, Criqui MH, *et al.* Preventing heart attack and death in patients with coronary disease. *Circulation* 1995; **92**: 2–4.

5   Pate RR, Pratt M, Blair SN, *et al.* Physical activity and public health. A recommendation from the Centers for Disease Control and Prevention and the American College of Sports Medicine. *JAMA* 1995; **273**: 402–7.

6   Nixon HL. Getting over the worry hurdle: parental encouragement and the sports involvement of visually impaired children and youths. *Adapt Phys Activ Quart* 1988; **5**: 29–43.

7 Block ME, Zeman R. Including students with disabilities in regular physical education: effects on nondisabled children. *Adapt Phys Activ Quart* 1996; **13**: 38–49.

8 Hoffman MD. Cardiorespiratory fitness and training in quadriplegics and paraplegics. *Sports Med* 1986; **3**: 312–30.

9 Bar Or O, Ward DS, Smith K, Longmuir P. *The use of Rating of Perceived Exertion for Exercise Prescription in Wheelchair-bound Children and Young Adults.* Toronto: Ontario Ministry of Tourism and Recreation, 1989.

10 O'Connell DG, Barnhart R, Parks L. Muscular endurance and wheelchair propulsion in children with cerebral palsy or myelomeningocele. *Arch Phys Med Rehabil* 1992; **73**: 709–11.

11 Bergman AB, Stamm SJ. The morbidity of cardiac nondisease in school children. *N Engl J Med* 1967; **276**: 1008–13.

12 Pueschel SM. Should children with Down syndrome be screened for atlantoaxial instability? *Arch Pediatr Adolesc Med* 1998; **152**: 123–5.

13 Webborn ADJ. Heat-related problems for the Paralympic Games, Atlanta 1996. *Br J Ther Rehabil* 1996; **3**: 429–36.

14 Curtis KA, McClanahan S, Hall KM, *et al.* Health, vocational, and functional status in spinal cord injured athletes and nonathletes. *Arch Phys Med Rehabil* 1986; **67**: 862–5.

15 Stotts KM. Health maintenance: paraplegic athletes and nonathletes. *Arch Phys Med Rehabil* 1986; **67**: 109–14.

16 Cooper RA, Quatrano LA, Axelson PW, *et al.* Research on physical activity and health among people with disabilities: a consensus statement. *J Rehabil Res Dev* 1999; **36**: 142–54.

Further reading

Fallon KE. The disabled athlete. In: Bloomfield J, Fricker PA, Fitch KD (eds). *Science and Medicine in Sport.* Carlton: Blackwell Science, 1995.

Goldberg B. *Sports and Exercise for Children with Chronic Health Conditions.* Champaign: Human Kinetics, 1995.

Webborn ADJ. Sport and disability. In: McLatchie G, Harries M, Williams C, King J (eds). *ABC of Sports Medicine 2e.* London: BMJ Publishing, 2000.

12 | Delivering an exercise prescription for patients with chronic fatigue

Richard Budgett

Introduction

Chronic fatigue and underperformance in athletes have much in common with chronic fatigue syndrome (CFS) in non athletic patients. When athletes fail to recover from training they become progressively fatigued and suffer from prolonged underperformance. They may also suffer from frequent minor infections (particularly respiratory infections). In the absence of any other medical cause, this is called unexplained underperformance syndrome (UPS), and in the past has been called overtraining syndrome, burnout, staleness or sports fatigue syndrome.[1-3] The condition is normally secondary to the stress of training but the exact aetiology and pathophysiology is unknown, and many factors other than overtraining may lead to failure to recover from training or competition.

Definitions

In athletes UPS is diagnosed when underperformance does not resolve despite two weeks of adequate rest and there is no other identifiable medical cause. Underperformance is normally accompanied by fatigue and an unexpected sense of effort. This contrasts with the definition of CFS, where symptoms must last at least six months.[4]

The normal response to training

All athletes, and any individual who exercises hard, will initially fatigue and underperform but if recovery is allowed, there is supercompensation and improvement in performance.[5] This is the theory of training. During the hard training or 'overload' period, transient symptoms and signs and changes in diagnostic tests may occur; this is called over-reaching.[6]

Over-reaching is associated with changes in the profile of mood state (POMS) questionnaire which shows reduced vigour and increased tension, depression, anger, fatigue and confusion.[7] Muscle glycogen stores are depleted and resting heart rate rises.[8] The testosterone/cortisol ratio is reduced due to lower testosterone and high cortisol levels. Microscopic damage to muscle also leads to raised creatine kinase levels if there is eccentric exercise.[9]

All these changes are physiological and normal if recovery occurs within two weeks (and it normally occurs within 24 hours). Over-reaching is a vital part of training for improved performance.[5] The question is whether training and exercise can be used to improve performance in someone who is chronically fatigued.

Abnormal response to training leading to chronic fatigue

This is best represented graphically (Fig 1). It is essential that any exercise programme does not make symptoms worse rather than better. The cyclical nature of most training programmes (periodisation) allows this recovery and full benefit from hard exercise.[10]

Symptoms of underperformance syndrome

The main complaint is of underperformance. Athletes will often ignore fatigue, heavy muscles and depression until performance is chronically affected.[11] Sleep disturbance occurs in over 90% of cases; with difficulty in getting to sleep, nightmares, waking in the night and waking

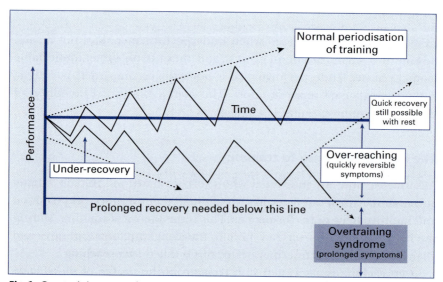

Fig 1. Overtraining or under-recovery, leading to the overtraining syndrome.

unrefreshed.[12] There may also be loss of appetite, weight loss, loss of competitive drive and libido and increased emotional lability, anxiety and irritability. The athlete may report a raised resting pulse rate and excessive sweating. Upper respiratory tract infections (URTI) or other minor infections frequently recur every time an athlete tries to return to training when they have not fully recovered. This gives an apparent cycle of recurrent infection every few weeks (Fig 2).[1,13,14] These symptoms are very similar to those of CFS.[4]

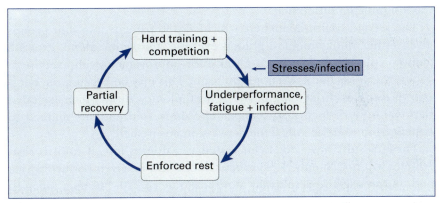

Fig 2. The cycle of recurrent minor infections.

Management

Athletes suffering from chronic fatigue and underperformance are different from sedentary individuals with CFS; because the athletes present earlier, they tend to recover more quickly, and there is an opportunity to alter the major stress in their lives (training and competition). Nevertheless, management is fundamentally similar for any individual with chronic fatigue and requires a holistic approach. Rest and regeneration strategies are central to recovery.[1,15]

Exercise therapy in chronic fatigue patients

If an exercise regimen (training programme) can improve performance in healthy individuals it is reasonable to hope that the same may be true in patients with CFS – be they athletes or not. CFS patients are certainly less physically fit probably due to deconditioning from resting.[16]

There have been two trials to test this hypothesis. The first was at St Bartholomew's Hospital and the National Sports Medicine Institute.[17]

After exclusions (depression or sleep disturbance) 66 patients entered the trial and were randomly allocated to exercise or flexibility groups and seen weekly for 12 weeks. Those in the exercise group were encouraged to exercise 5 times per week at a very low level, using a heart rate monitor. The duration of each exercise session was increased individually on a weekly basis from 10 mins initially up to a maximum of 30 mins per day after which intensity was increased. There were very few drop outs. Sixteen of the 29 (55%) who completed the exercise programme rated themselves as much better or very much better compared to 8 of the 30 who completed the flexibility treatment. This was a significant difference.

The second trial in Manchester divided 136 patients into four groups given either fluoxetine and graded exercise, fluoxetine alone, exercise alone or placebo.[18] There was a trend for improvement with exercise at 12 and 24 weeks but it was not significant. This may be because the entry criteria were less strict than for the St Bartholomew's trial which excluded depression and sleep disturbance. The depressed patients seemed to benefit from exercise only if the depression was treated.

These results have not been tested in athletes but, if told to rest, athletes will not comply.[15,19] So they, too, should be given positive advice and told to exercise aerobically at a pulse rate of 120–140 bpm for 5–10 min each day, ideally in divided sessions, and slowly build this up over 6–12 weeks. The exercise programme has to be individually designed and depends on the clinical picture and rate of improvement. The cycle of partial recovery followed by hard training and recurrent breakdown needs to be stopped. It is often necessary to avoid the athlete's own sport using cross training, because of the tendency to increase the exercise intensity too quickly. A positive approach is essential, with an emphasis on slowly building up volume rather than intensity to about one hour per day. Once this volume is tolerated, then more intensive work can be incorporated, above the onset of blood lactate accumulation (OBLA).[19] Progress can be monitored by performance and symptoms using a self-administered questionnaire and visual analogue scales.[20,21]

Sprint and power athletes never seem to break down with UPS in the same way as endurance athletes, probably because of the large amounts of rest incorporated into their programmes.[22] Thus, another form of exercise has been added to the rehabilitation programme. Very short (less than 10s) sprints or power exercises with at least 3–5 min of rest appear safe and allow some hard training to be done. The athletes do this session 2–3 times per week.[23]

Athletes who have been underperforming for many months are often surprised at the good performance they can produce after 12 weeks of extremely light exercise. At this point, care must be taken not to increase the intensity of training too fast and also to allow full recovery after hard parts of their training cycle. It is recommended that athletes recover completely at least once a week and regularly have light periods in a carefully periodised programme.[24]

Conclusion

The unexplained UPS affects mainly endurance athletes. It is a condition of underperformance and chronic fatigue with an increased vulnerability to infection leading to recurrent infections. It is not yet known how the stress of hard training and competition contributes to the observed spectrum of symptoms. With a very careful exercise regimen and regeneration strategies symptoms normally resolve in 6–12 weeks but may continue much longer or recur if athletes return to hard training too soon.

Patients with CFS present a similar picture to athletes with UPS but by definition the problem has lasted for at least six months. Recovery, although helped by a twelve-week exercise programme, normally takes far longer than in athletes. There is evidence that a graded exercise programme is an effective treatment strategy for patients with CFS. It will help many, and the studies reassure us that it will do no harm. There is no place for bed rest in the treatment of these patients.

References

1 Budgett R. The overtraining syndrome. *Br Med J* 1994; **309**: 4465–8.
2 Fry RW, Morton AR, Keast D. Overtraining syndrome and the chronic fatigue syndrome. *NZ J Sports Med* 1991; **19**: 48–52.
3 Lehmann M, Foster C, Keull J. Overtraining in endurance athletes: a brief review. *Med Sci Sports Exerc* 1993; **25**: 854–62.
4 Royal College of Physicians. *Chronic Fatigue Syndrome: Report of a Joint Working Group of the Royal Colleges of Physicians, Psychiatrists and General Practitioners.* London: Royal College of Physicians, 1996.
5 Morton RH. Modelling training and overtraining. *J Sports Sci* 1997; **15**: 335–40.
6 Budgett R. The overtraining syndrome. *Br J Sports Med* 1990; **24**: 231–6.
7 Morgan WP, Costill DC, Flynn MG, *et al.* Mood disturbance following increased training in swimmers. *Med Sci Sporst Exerc* 1988; **20**: 408–14.
8 Costill DL, Flynn MG, Kirway JP, *et al.* Effects of repeated days of intensified training on muscle glycogen and swimming performance. *Med Sci Sports Exerc* 1988; **20**: 249–54.
9 Schwane JA, Williams JS, Sloan JH. Effects of training on delayed muscle soreness and serum creatine kinase activity after running. *Med Sci Sports Exerc* 1987; **19**: 584–90.
10 Fry RW, Morton AR, Keast D. Periodisation and the prevention of over-training. *Can J Sports Sci* 1992; **17**: 241–8.

11   Dyment P. Frustrated by chronic fatigue? *Physician Sports Med* 1993; **21**: 47–54.

12   Koutedakis Y, Budgett R, Faulmann L. Rest in underperforming elite competitors. *Br J Sports Med* 1990; **24**: 248–52. `

13   Nieman D, Johanssen LM, Lee JW, Arabatzis K. Infections episodes before and after the Los Angeles Marathon. *J Sports Med Phys Fitness* 1990; **30**: 289–96.

14   Nieman D. Exercise infection and immunity. *Int J Sports Med* 1994; **15**: S131.

15   Smith C, Kirby P, Noakes TD. The worn-out athlete: A clinical approach to chronic fatigue in athletes. *J Sports Sci* 1997; **15**: 341–51.

16   Saltin B, Bloomquist G, Mitchell J, *et al.* Response to exercise after bedrest and after training. *Circulation* 1968; **38**: S1–55.

17   Fulcher KY, White PD. Randomised controlled trial of graded exercise in patients with the chronic fatigue syndrome. *Br Med J* 1997; **314**: 1647–52.

18   Wearden AJ, Morris RK, Mullis R, *et al.* A randomised, double blind, placebo controlled treatment trial of fluoxetine and a graded exercise programme for chronic fatigue syndrome. *Br J Psychiatry* 1998; **172**: 485–90.

19   Budgett R. The overtraining syndrome. *Coaching Focus* 1995; **28**: 4–6.

20   Morgan WP, Brown DR, Raglin JS, *et al.* Psychological monitoring of overtraining and staleness. *Br J Sports Med* 1987; **21**: 107–14.

21   Hooper SL, Mackinnon LT. Monitoring overtraining in athletes. *Sports Med* 1995; **20**: 231–7.

22   Fry AC, Kraemer WJ. Does short-term near-maximal intensity machine resistance training induce overtraining? *J Strength Conditioning Res* 1994; **8**: 188–91.

23   Budgett R. Fatigue and underperformance in athletes: the overtraining syndrome. *Br Med J* 1998; **32**: 107–10.

24   Morton RH. The quantitative periodisation of athletic training: a model study. *Sports Med: Training Rehabil* 1991; **3**: 19–28.

13 | The future: the clinical exercise practitioner

Bob Laventure

Introduction

The promotion of physical activity (defined as 'any bodily movement produced by the contraction of skeletal muscle that substantially increases energy expenditure'[1]) as a valid public health intervention was given a high public and professional profile in the UK through the former Health Education Authority's national campaign *Active for life*. The promotion of physical activity of a moderate intensity on most days of the week[2] is exemplified by the range of new walking programmes such as the British Heart Foundation and Countryside Agency partnership *Walking the way to health*,[3] and the promotion of health related cycling schemes.[4,5]

The promotion of exercise (physical activity that is 'planned, structured, and repetitive bodily movement done to improve or maintain one or more of the components of physical fitness'[1]) has been associated with the growth of interest in aerobic activities such as jogging and exercise classes and, through the exercise and fitness industry, with the growth of fitness and health centres.

A more recent development has been in the use of exercise as a specific form of intervention to meet a range of health needs, eg to target those at risk from ischaemic heart disease. This has resulted in the development and expansion of exercise referral schemes in primary healthcare.[6]

More recently still, supported by an increase in research activity, there has been increased interest in the potential role of exercise for the treatment of patients with certain clinical conditions, eg diabetes, arthritis and hypertension, much of which has built on models of practice developed in cardiac rehabilitation.

This chapter will outline corresponding developments in the knowledge, skills, training and professionalisation of the exercise instructor which have resulted in the emergence of the clinical exercise practitioner as a respected member of the interdisciplinary, secondary healthcare team.

Standards among exercise practitioners

Until fairly recently, training and education of the exercise instructor was delivered largely through training organisations within the fitness and exercise industry. Continuing professional development was delivered through governing bodies and commercial fitness organisations. Most instructors had been trained to work with motivated, relatively healthy and mostly young people. In the last ten years however, an increasing number have undertaken training in exercise for special populations, eg exercise for the older person, or exercise for ante- and post-natal women. Nevertheless, the emphasis in all these modules was still very much on low risk, relatively healthy individuals. Then came the growth of exercise referral schemes, first in primary health care[7] and later with additional targeted patient groups.[8] These highlighted the need for additional development of the training continuum, in recognition of the greater skills, knowledge and understanding required of the exercise practitioner.

In 1998, Exercise England (then the governing body for exercise in England) undertook a review of the qualifications and competencies relating to exercise programming, based on criteria developed by the National Training Organisation for Sport, Recreation and Allied Occupations (SPRITO). The purpose was to define competencies and standards in coaching, leading and teaching in sport and exercise. The present situation, as described in the National Quality Assurance Framework (see below), is summarised in Table 1. The table matches participant characteristics with exercise professionals' expertise, in the context of the UK National Occupational Standards (NOS). It also facilitates progression both within and between areas of competence, eg as described in *Exercise for Improving Postural Stability and Reducing the Risk of Falls and Injuries.*[10]

The National Quality Assurance Framework for Exercise Referral Systems[9] was commissioned by the Department of Health and developed by the British Association of Sports and Exercise Sciences (BASES) and Exercise England. It sets out guidelines for the competencies required of the exercise practitioner in the primary health care setting, with corresponding indicators. Examples of these are shown in Box 1.

The publication and dissemination of this document have been important steps. The next objectives must be to ensure its wholehearted implementation, and to develop an equivalent quality assurance framework for services in secondary care.

The National Exercise and Fitness Register

The National Quality Assurance Framework recommends professional registration of exercise practitioners as a pre-requisite for working in

Table 1. The exercise professional's level of expertise is matched with participant characteristics (Adapted from ref [9])

Title	NOS Level	Client group	Activity	Predominant Source
Exercise & Fitness Coach, Teacher, Instructor	2	Very low risk. Apparently healthy, mostly motivated and paying customers	Includes exercise to music, weight- and circuit-training	Self-referral and primary care recommendation
Advanced Instructor (Referred Populations-1) ('Exercise Practitioner')	3	Low risk, eg older people, pre- and post-natal women.	Exercise adaptations required	Primary care referral
Advanced Instructor (Referred Populations-2) ('Exercise Practitioner')	3	Medium risk. People with specific chronic diseases and disabilities (eg community-based cardiac, falls or osteoporosis rehabilitation)	Exercise specific and adapted to meet needs of the individual and their specific condition(s)	Primary care referral
Advanced Instructor (Clinical Exercise) ('Clinical Exercise Practitioner')	3 plus extra training	Significant health risk. People with specific chronic diseases and disabilities (eg hospital-based cardiac, falls or osteoporosis rehabilitation)	Exercise specific and adapted to meet needs of the individual and their specific condition(s). Delivered in close collaboration with other health professionals.	Secondary care referral.

NOS=National Occupational Standards.

primary health care settings. The Professional Register for Exercise and Fitness (England), supported by Sport England and operated by the Fitness Industry Association (FIA) under the auspices of SPRITO provides the check on qualifications, a code of ethics and professional conduct, as well as a system for complaints and disciplinary action. It also outlines requirements for continuing professional development and other quality control mechanisms required of exercise instructors working in exercise referral settings. In short, it provides the means of self-regulation of the exercise industry in line with other professional bodies and sets standards for safety and effectiveness for the protection and information of clients/patients, referrers, local authorities and health authorities. Similar systems for registration of instructors exist in Scotland and Wales.

Box 1
Examples of guidelines and indicators for the competencies required of the exercise practitioner: (Adapted from ref [9])

▶ *Guideline 1:* Instructors delivering supervised exercise will hold appropriate qualifications and insurance and will follow standards of practice, a code of ethics and guidelines of accountability, and possess a current first aid award which includes a cardio-pulmonary resuscitation award.

Indicator: The exercise instructor is included on the Professional Register for Exercise and Fitness (England) at the appropriate level and is engaged in continuing professional development, part of which must relate to the competencies required to carry out their role in the referral scheme.

▶ *Guideline 2:* Instructors should understand and apply a proven model of behaviour change in interactions with referred patients participating in the referral scheme.

Indicator: Successful completion of training in skills and strategies that support best practice for motivational skills and strategies for facilitating exercise behaviour change and evidence of application in practice.

▶ *Guideline 4:* Instructors should understand the efficacy of physical activity in relation to likely health gains and/or the management of specific medical conditions.

Indicator: Instructors will be able to demonstrate an understanding of the possible implications of referred conditions and medications on the exercise response and physical activity capability. They will be able to demonstrate the ability to design exercise programmes with special considerations relating to the comfort and safety of the referred patient.

▶ *Guideline 7:* A health and physical activity history should be taken by the exercise instructor and confirmed against the information from the referrer, etc.

Indicator: Evidence of a completed health and physical activity history for each patient will be on file together with a date stamped note of any further contact with the referrer.

Exercise in the secondary care setting

In the secondary care setting the patient's needs are identified and met by the combined skills and experiences of an interdisciplinary professional team delivering a holistic care plan. For example, cardiac rehabilitation programmes include education and advice on smoking cessation, diet and physical activity.[11] Similarly, falls prevention and management programmes for older people which involve exercise are most effective when they also include modification of other risk factors, such as polypharmacy, vision problems and environmental hazards.[12]

Working as part of such a team, the clinical exercise practitioner is required to collaborate with other health professionals and provide evidence-based exercise interventions, participate in patient and programme review, and provide continuity between secondary care and the community exercise setting.

The variable health status of patients with specific diseases and conditions demands a highly individualised approach to exercise and exercise referral which will have safety and effectiveness as key requirements. In order to work effectively with patients who have little or no previous experience of physical activity or exercise and who may well have very poor motivation to undertake an exercise programme, the clinical exercise practitioner will need to employ proven models of patient counselling and readiness to change.

Providing continuity and sustaining exercise behaviour

Continuity between the supervised programme delivered in the secondary care setting and measures to sustain long-term participation in a community exercise setting are essential elements of long-term patient care. Providing such continuity will:

i   assist in optimising the gains achieved in the secondary healthcare setting
ii provide a mechanism for referral back to the health setting in the event of a decline in health
iii increase the likelihood of long-term adherence to regular exercise.

Exercise referral in secondary healthcare and professional responsibility

Just as in primary healthcare settings, clinical responsibility rests with the referrer. It is implicit, therefore, that only a medically qualified individual, or another health professional working within a protocol with delegated authority, can initiate a referral to an exercise referral scheme.

Responsibility for the administration, design and delivery of the programme, on the other hand, rests with the clinical exercise practitioner service. To take this share of the overall responsibility, those supervising the conduct of the exercise must be able to demonstrate that they have been appropriately trained.

The role of the clinical exercise practitioner

Clinical exercise practitioners are able to work in a number of specialist settings and environments, including the physiotherapy gym, hospital ward, day hospital, specialist rehabilitation unit and nursing home. As Advanced Exercise Instructors they acquired the skills, experience, competencies and qualifications to:

i understand patient motivation, eg readiness to change, barriers that might prevent exercise and attitudes towards exercise (including, for example, the concerns of some older or disabled people that exercise might do more harm than good[13])

ii adapt and modify the exercise programme to ensure it is safe and effective, taking account of the individual patient's needs and vulnerabilities

iii work with the particular limitations of special population groups (eg older people, people with disabilities or stable chronic health problems) where the accompanying health risk is low.

In addition, in order to deliver exercise to people requiring a more specific or 'prescriptive' approach and where the accompanying health risk is moderate (eg community-based ('phase IV') cardiac rehabilitation, community-based falls prevention, mild to moderate depression, HIV positive health scheme), the Advanced Instructor (Referred Populations-2) will have undertaken additional training. This will have included details of the disease specific to the clinical service, its complications, its medications and their implications for exercise. For example, the British Association of Cardiac Rehabilitation (BACR) Phase IV training module[14] and the DoH-funded Exercise for the Prevention of Falls and Injuries training module[10] are the recognised standards for insuring advanced instructors working at this level. Such further training will be reflected in the exercise instructor's entry in the Professional Register for Exercise and Fitness. Other modules at this advanced level are currently in development or have been proposed, including Exercise and Mental Health, Osteoporosis and Arthritis Care.

The Advanced Instructor (Clinical Exercise), or 'clinical exercise practitioner', will have undertaken yet further additional training, provided or recommended by the leader of their interdisciplinary secondary healthcare team. They will have a greater depth of knowledge and understanding of the clinical conditions encountered in their particular sphere of practice. The details of the clinical exercise practitioner's precise role and responsibilities will be influenced by the clinical condition of the patients, the skill mix of the interdisciplinary team, and the previous professional background of the practitioner.

Opportunities for expansion and development

Much of the role of the clinical exercise practitioner has been pioneered through the experience of those working in cardiac rehabilitation teams. However, recent guidance for the role of exercise in the prevention and management of falls[12,15] and for mental health[8] suggests that there is significant potential for the expansion of the role of the clinical exercise practitioner.

To ensure adherence to the criteria and quality standards of safety, evidence and effectiveness, further developments must be guided by the same four key principles that have underpinned progress to date. These are:

1. The starting point should be an evidence based review and expert consensus to inform the exercise programme design.
2. Agreed evidence based protocols and guidelines for interventions should be established.
3. Curriculum development should be followed by pilot courses which are closely monitored and evaluated.
4. Training courses should be nationally available with mechanisms in place to ensure quality control, maintenance of standards and responsiveness to the publication of new evidence.

Collaboration between exercise and health professionals

Much of the knowledge and experience required to develop further curricula and training for the clinical exercise practitioner has already been acquired, but has yet to be translated into accessible education opportunities and practice. In some cases the necessary leadership in this process may come from high-profile, disease-specific organisations. In others, it may come from special interest groups within the health professions. It may also be led by local health partnerships and alliances working in specific communities, hospital units or specialist centres.

As yet, however, no single, national health or exercise organisation has stepped forward to take responsibility for the recognition and dissemination of these developments in the UK. In the USA, this role has been taken by the American College of Sports Medicine (ACSM), but its authoritative guidance on the management of persons with specific clinical exercise needs[16] cannot necessarily be applied directly to the UK. An equivalent British initiative is required. Future developments that intend to establish the work of the clinical exercise practitioner will depend upon new forms of collaboration among a range of health and exercise professionals, perhaps in partnership with organisations such as the National Institute for Clinical Excellence (NICE) in England and the Scottish Intercollegiate Guideline Network.

Looking to the future – recommendations

To ensure that future exercise initiatives meet the wide range of needs identified above and also meet the quality standards and expectations of government health agendas, development of the role of the clinical exercise practitioner should include the following five aspects:

1. Additional curriculum development, providing nationally validated and accessible protocols, guidelines and education and training programmes.
2. A career development route for the clinical exercise practitioner which respects many different professional backgrounds and starting points.
3. Formulation of the practical competencies for best exercise practice in secondary healthcare, which go beyond those developed for the primary care setting.
4. Greater collaboration at national and local levels between medical and exercise professionals.
5. Medical professional support for the Professional Register for Exercise and Fitness (England) and its counterparts in the other countries of the UK.

Acknowledgements

The author wishes to acknowledge the contributions of Susie Dinan and Andrew Craig with comments on drafts of this paper.

References

1   US Department of Health and Human Services. *Physical Activity and Health: a Report of the Surgeon General.* Atlanta, GA: US Department of Health and

Human Services, Centers for Disease Control and Prevention, National Center for Chronic Disease Prevention and Health Promotion, 1996.

2 Department of Health. *More People, More Active, More Often. Physical Activity in England – a Consultation Paper*. London: Department of Health, 1995.

3 Countryside Agency. *Practical Guidelines for Developing Walking for Health*. Cheltenham: Countryside Agency, 1999.

4 British Medical Association. *Road Transport and Health*, London: BMA, 1997.

5 Department of the Environment, Transport and the Regions. *National Cycling Forum, Promoting Cycling, Improving Health*. London: DETR, 1999.

6 Riddoch C, Puig-Ribera A, Cooper A. *Effectiveness of Physical Activity promotion Schemes in Primary Health Care: A Review. Health Promotion Effectiveness Reviews No 14*. London: Health Education Authority, 1998.

7 Harland J, White M, Drinkwater C, *et al.* The Newcastle exercise project: a randomised controlled trial of methods to promote physical activity in primary care. *BMJ* 1999; **319**: 828–32.

8 Department of Health. *Physical Activity and Mental Health. Guidelines for Local Practice*. London: Department of Health, 2000.

9 Department of Health. *Exercise Referral Systems: a National Quality Assurance Framework*. London: The Stationery Office, 2001.

10 Dinan S, Skelton D (eds). *Exercise for Improving Postural Stability and Reducing the Risk of Falls and Injuries. A Specialist Training Course for Health and Exercise Professionals*. Leicester: Leicester College, 2000.

11 Bell J. *Delivering an exercise prescription for patients with coronary artery disease*. In: Young A, Harris M (eds). *Physical Activity for Patients: an Exercise Prescription*. London: Royal College of Physicians, 2001.

12 Queen Mary and Westfield College and South East Institute of Public Health. *Guidelines for the Prevention of Falls in Older People*. London: Department of Health, 1998.

13 Finch H. *Physical Activity 'At Our Age'. Qualitative Research Among People Over the Age of 50*. London: Health Education Authority, 1997.

14 Bell J (ed). *Phase IV Exercise Instructor Training (2e)*. London: British Association for Cardiac Rehabilitation, 2000.

15 Health Education Authority. *Physical Activity and the Prevention and Management of Falls among Older People – a Framework for Practice*. London: Health Education Authority, 1999.

16 American College of Sports Medicine. *ACSM's Exercise Management for Persons with Chronic Disease and Disabilities*. Champaign, Illinios: Human Kinetics, 1997.

14 | The future: specialist training in sport and exercise medicine in the UK and Ireland

Donald A D Macleod

Introduction

Sport and exercise medicine is at the threshold of exciting developments in the UK and Ireland. The medical profession will soon be able to meet the legitimate expectations of exercisers, sports participants and governing bodies of sport for advice about prevention, treatment and rehabilitation of sports injuries and illnesses, and the use of exercise to minimise or enhance recovery from a wide range of clinical problems.

Postgraduate educational opportunities are already available to doctors who wish to develop their professional interest in sport and exercise. In 1998, the Academy of Medical Royal Colleges acknowledged public and professional expectations by establishing the Intercollegiate Academic Board of Sport and Exercise Medicine. The board is responsible to its parent colleges and faculties for setting, appraising and developing basic and higher specialist training programmes in sport and exercise medicine, mirroring the standards required by all currently established specialties in British and Irish medicine.

The final step in the development of the specialty will be the provision of jobs in academic and NHS practice, by governing bodies of sports, by national and regional institutes of sport and professional sports clubs or associations. In every respect, progress is being made.

Background

The provision of medical services for individuals taking regular exercise or while participating in sport has traditionally been patchy in the UK and Ireland. Doctors had limited access to appropriate training or educational opportunities and there were virtually no paid jobs. Medical services for sport and exercise medicine were invariably provided by interested individuals, occasionally within their normal clinical practice but usually on a voluntary basis. Many of these individuals were current or previous participants in sport and were 'giving something back'.

Governing bodies and sport coaches have always regarded medical involvement in sport with suspicion. These organisations and individuals were concerned that doctors would try to neuter their sport by attempting to introduce changes to minimise potential injury. Gradually, this climate has changed, and governing bodies, coach education programmes and clubs have recognised the positive contribution that sports medicine can make with regard to the safety and development of their sport.

Individual athletes and sports participants have also regarded the medical profession with suspicion. Unfortunately, their attitude was based on doctors' indifference to and ignorance of exercise physiology and the management of soft tissue injuries. In addition, the greater part of the medical profession considered that doctors involved in sports medicine, other than the occasional orthopaedic surgeon, were wasting their time or were only there for the 'gin and tonic'. This negative attitude in the medical profession delayed and prevented interest in the benefits of exercise as a relevant component in the management of a wide range of clinical conditions and as an essential part of a healthy lifestyle.

Exercisers and sports participants have gradually come to realise that the medical profession can make a positive contribution to the prevention and management of sports injuries, to a physically active lifestyle and to the role of exercise in the management of disability or rehabilitation from illness.

Educational opportunities

The British Association of Sport and Medicine was established in 1954 by Lord Arthur Porritt and Sir Adolphe Abraham, who were both doctors and former Olympic athletes. This multidisciplinary organisation, which recently changed its name to the British Association of Sport and Exercise Medicine (BASEM), has developed an integrated programme of introductory, intermediate and master class educational courses and conferences on a national and regional basis. BASEM also established the *British Journal of Sports Medicine* (currently published by BMJ Publications), which has an excellent reputation and is increasingly recognised internationally as one of the leading journals in the field of sport and exercise medicine.

The Royal Society of Medicine established a Sports Medicine section in 1993.

In addition, some universities in the UK and Ireland have developed taught degree courses (MSc) on a full or part time basis (Box 1). Many of these courses are open to graduates from the professions allied to medicine as well as to doctors.

The UK and English Sports Councils combined in 1992 to establish a

---

Box 1
Taught MSc Courses in Sports Medicine:

► Royal London Hospital, London

► Queen's Medical Centre, University of Nottingham

► Department of continuing and distance learning, University of Bath

► Institute of biomedical and life sciences, University of Glasgow

► Department of anatomy, Trinity College, Dublin

► School of health sciences, Leeds Metropolitan University

► Faculty of Education and Sport, University of Wales Institute

► Royal Free and University College Medical School, London

National Sports Medicine Institute of the UK (NSMI). This organisation collates information regarding all educational programmes available to the medical profession. In addition, NSMI administers the educational programme developed by BASEM.

The three ancient Scottish medical Royal Colleges (The Royal College of Surgeons of Edinburgh, the Royal College of Physicians of Edinburgh and the Royal College of Physicians and Surgeons of Glasgow) established a Diploma examination in sport and exercise medicine in 1989. The three Colleges had agreed, following the 13th Commonwealth Games (held in Edinburgh in 1986), to develop a syllabus which would act as the basis for identifying someone who could safely be described as a 'touchline doctor'. The essential features of the syllabus covered a wide range of relevant basic sciences with regard to exercise physiology and anatomy as well as acknowledging the role of exercise in the promotion of health. The syllabus also covered the wide ranging aspects of illness and injury that can be encountered on an everyday basis among exercisers and sports participants. The exam tested the life saving skills of the doctor should he or she be present when a sports participant or exerciser might collapse or be seriously injured. The Society of Apothecaries of London also developed a Diploma Examination in Sports Medicine in 1989. This Diploma included a case report and dissertation as well as oral and clinical components.

The combination of BASEM educational programmes, the *British Journal of Sports Medicine*, the Royal Society of Medicine section, the Scottish Royal Colleges and Society of Apothecaries Diploma examinations in Sports Medicine, the taught MSc degree courses and the Bath distance learning programme have produced a cohort of motivated, well educated and committed doctors, prepared to offer the highest standards of medical practice to their patients as well as the community at large, exercisers and sports participants.

Standards of practice

During the 1990s, a series of publications and developments took place, recognising the importance of exercise and sport to the community at large. In addition, the government became increasingly concerned to promote excellence in sport. It was recognised that these developments (Box 2) would inevitably increase the demands made of the medical profession.

Box 2
Sports medicine – the political agenda

▶ Medical aspects of exercise – benefits and risks
  Royal College of Physicians of London, 1991
▶ TOYA and sports injuries
  The Sports Council, London, 1992
▶ National fitness survey
  Allied Dunbar, 1992
▶ Exercise, health, benefits and risks
  European Occupational Health Series No 7, 1993
▶ Sport and exercise medicine – policy and provision
  British Medical Association, 1996
▶ Sport raising the game
  Department of National Heritage, 1995
▶ A sporting future for all
  Department for Culture, Media and Sports, 2000

Standards of clinical practice in any specialty are set, appraised and developed by the medical Royal Colleges and their faculties. The Specialist Training Authority (STA) approves training programmes undertaken by doctors who are then registered as specialists by the General Medical Council (GMC).

Currently, sport and exercise medicine is not recognised as a specialty in the UK and Ireland. Recognition of a new specialty is a complex process involving the STA and the NHS Executive Medical Education

Unit before the Secretary of State will give approval to amend the relevant schedule.

Following a series of working parties and extended discussions, the Academy of Medical Royal Colleges (AMRC) agreed that interested Royal Colleges and Faculties could establish, in April 1998, the Intercollegiate Academic Board of Sport and Exercise Medicine (IABSEM) (Box 3). This board was charged with the responsibility of establishing a unified training programme in sport and exercise medicine for the UK and Ireland based on appropriate educational and training programmes and diploma examinations.

The initial activities of the Board have been directed to reviewing the syllabus and examinations of the Scottish Medical Royal Colleges and Society of Apothecaries, incorporating them into a new Diploma for Sport and Exercise Medicine for the UK and Ireland. This Diploma continues to assess the 'touchline doctor' and is equivalent to the basic

---

Box 3
Membership of the Intercollegiate Academic Board for Sport and Exercise Medicine

- ▶ Royal College of Surgeons of Edinburgh
- ▶ Royal College of Physicians of Edinburgh
- ▶ Royal College of Physicians and Surgeons of Glasgow
- ▶ Royal College of Surgeons of England
- ▶ Royal College of Physicians of London
- ▶ Royal College of Surgeons of Ireland
- ▶ Royal College of Physicians of Ireland
- ▶ Royal College of General Practitioners
- ▶ Royal College of Pathologists
- ▶ Royal College of Radiologists
- ▶ Royal College of Paediatrics and Child Health
- ▶ Royal College of Ophthalmologists
- ▶ Faculty of Dental Surgery, Royal College of Surgeons, England
- ▶ Faculty of Occupational Medicine
- ▶ Faculty of Public Health Medicine

Associate Members
- ▶ Faculty of Accident and Emergency Medicine
- ▶ Medical Services of the Armed Forces
- ▶ Society of Apothecaries of London

specialty training exams undertaken by a wide range of currently established specialties such as medicine, surgery, paediatrics, anaesthetics, etc.

IABSEM has recently received approval from the Academy of Medical Royal Colleges to develop higher specialty training programmes for a small number of doctors in sport and exercise medicine. IABSEM would expect the current Diploma examination to be an entry criterion for higher specialty training in this field.

Specialty training opportunities

Specialty training in the UK and Ireland has changed in recent years with the introduction of Calman training programmes (Box 4). Medical graduates spend one year as a pre-registration House Officer before they are registered by the GMC and move into what is a minimum two-year general professional and basic specialty training programme. At that stage, young doctors must choose whether they wish to train in general practice, hospital medicine or aspects of community health. The duration of these higher or more specialised training programmes vary from a minimum of one year in general practice to a range of 4–6 years in hospital or community medicine.

IABSEM believes that doctors should be able to prepare themselves for the Diploma examination in sport and exercise medicine and meet all the syllabus requirements as part of their general professional and basic specialty training.

Box 4
UK and Ireland medical training

House Officer	1 year
Senior House Officer	2 years general professional/basic specialty training (minimum)

TIME TO CHOOSE A SPECIALTY

Specialist Registrar in:

General practice 1 year minimum training	Hospital specialties 4–6 years training	Community medicine 4–6 years training

The higher training of specialists in sport and exercise medicine will come under two categories. Doctors currently training as specialist registrars in a wide range of specialties are entitled to one year's leave of absence from their programme during which time they can undertake additional relevant training to broaden their experience. This training might include research but equally could extend to a structured one year higher training programme in Sport and Exercise Medicine. The Specialty Advisory Committees (SAC) which currently control the higher specialty training programmes for both rheumatology and rehabilitation medicine have already agreed that a one year flexible training programme in sport and exercise medicine will meet the flexible training requirements of doctors in these two specialties.

IABSEM hopes to extend this one year flexible training opportunity to a wide range of additional specialties by discussing their proposals with the relevant SACs. This would include community specialties, such as public health, health education or occupational medicine as well as general practice and hospital specialties such as accident and emergency medicine, paediatrics and child health, respiratory medicine, cardiology and orthopaedics.

IABSEM also hopes to develop four-year full time specialty training programmes in sport and exercise medicine to help meet the aspirations of the public and government, promoting exercise as an essential ingredient of a healthy lifestyle, as part of rehabilitation and as part of the management of a wide range of medical conditions. Doctors fully trained in sport and exercise medicine will also cater for the requirements of sports participants but particularly for athletes at the elite level.

The current university-based taught Masters degree courses may be considered suitable by SACs for one year of a specialist training programme. The identification of training centres and the approval of training programmes for a four year course in sport and exercise medicine will require close liaison with a wide range of bodies including the Conference of Postgraduate Medical Deans of the United Kingdom (COPMed). Potential sources of funding to meet the training requirements of this cohort of young doctors will have to be identified.

Tomorrow's world

If sport and exercise medicine is to develop in the UK, it will have to be an integrated, consultant-based specialty working in all aspects of the NHS, including hospital medicine, the community, primary care and the universities. Jobs are essential.

Sport will also need to provide paid posts on a part-time or full-time basis. Governing bodies, clubs, players unions and organisations such as the British Olympic Association and Commonwealth Games Association will need to recognise in financial terms the importance of specialist medical advice.

The British Government is currently developing a series of Institutes of Sport at UK, National and Regional levels to identify, promote and develop elite athletes. These organisations will require the very best specialist medical advice and they will need to liaise closely with academic and NHS medical services.

Doctors professing an interest in sport and exercise medicine will also have to ensure that they meet the requirements of continuing professional development in this aspect of their full time or part time medical practice. They will therefore have to include in their personal development portfolio membership of the relevant specialty association (BASEM) and evidence that they are continuing to participate in appropriate medical education and professional development courses. The annual appraisal and five-year revalidation programmes currently being discussed by the GMC will extend to cover all aspects of a doctor's clinical practice and this will, in the future, include sport and exercise medicine.

Conclusion

The benefits of exercise as an integral part of a healthy lifestyle, and as contributing positively to the treatment and rehabilitation of many medical and psychological conditions are well recognised. Promoting and prescribing exercise are accepted as professional skills that today's doctor should include in their clinical portfolio.

Non-competitive exercise should be risk free, but sport inevitably involves competition and risk which will lead to injuries and occasional illness, frequently at a significant cost to both the individual and society. Achieving excellence in sport requires considerable professional sports medicine support.

Currently, there are opportunities for medical practitioners to attend appropriate educational programmes to enhance their clinical portfolio. The flexible and full-time specialist training programmes being developed by the Intercollegiate Academic Board for Sport and Exercise Medicine are still in their infancy but hold great promise for the future.

Useful associations

Intercollegiate Academic Board of Sport and Exercise Medicine (IAMSEM), 6 Hill Square, Edinburgh EH8 9DR.

British Association of Sport and Exercise Medicine (BASEM). Registered office: 12 Greenside Avenue, Frodsham, Cheshire WA6 7SA.

The National Sports Medicine Institute of the United Kingdom (NSMI), c/o Medical College of St. Bartholomews Hospital, Charterhouse Square, London EC1M 6BQ.

The Royal Society of Medicine (RSM), Sports Medicine Section, 1 Wimpole Street, London W1M 8AE.

15 | The future: physical activity for all

Yvette Cooper MP

Introduction

The government recognises the important role of physical activity in health and is currently undergoing a long process of consultation in this area. This involves various meetings with, for example, the Modernisation Action Group and the Prevention and Inequalities Group, where discussions are held on improving performance across the NHS. Part of the government's National Plan for Health is, not only to increase the emphasis on prevention before people become ill and before people have any contact with the NHS, but also to increase the role of the NHS working in primary care, secondary care, local authorities, with other agencies such as local voluntary organisations and the leisure sector, and with the community, to shift the focus increasingly onto prevention.

Detailed negotiations are currently underway (between civil servants across departments and the Treasury in Whitehall) on targets, aims and new policies etc, which are all geared towards final announcements in July on what the main aims and targets are, and what it is the government needs to do. Unusually for health, we have had our announcement up front. We have the largest sustained increase in resources for health ever known: an annual average real terms growth rate of 6.3%. This is twice the historic growth rate.[1] However, the debate on how we spend it, and on what the priorities are, is effectively a public debate and we are trying to draw in as many people as possible to determine what those priorities should be. Therefore, as part of the Prevention and Inequalities Group, discussions are on issues around diet, smoking and exercise and also links with what Acheson called the 'upstream' causes of ill health, eg poverty, unemployment and housing.[2] It is particularly important because of our focus on three main disease areas as our priorities: coronary heart disease (CHD) and stroke, mental health and cancer. We have set a strong target for CHD and stroke in particular, to reduce the number of deaths over the next 10 years. Prevention is a strong part of that. We know that major chronic diseases such as CHD and stroke are largely preventable, however, they take a massive toll on individuals and society as a whole.

Heart disease is one of the biggest killers of men and women in the UK, and accounts for 115,000 deaths each year. Stroke is the leading cause of disability in the UK and the combined cost to the NHS is about £3.8 billion per year. Also importantly, these diseases affect people on lower incomes more significantly. The death rate from CHD among unskilled men is three times higher than among professional men, and this gap has widened over the past 20 years.[3]

The role of prevention in the National Service Framework (NSF) for CHD[4] and in work across the board is clearly considerable. The government has already set out a lot of action on anti-smoking, which is now being implemented across the country, both in terms of the increasing smoking cessation services (one week's free nicotine replacement therapy on prescription), and bans on tobacco advertising. Now the government is increasing its focus on other areas such as diet and exercise. There is a lot of work still to be done in terms of developing policies that will make a difference in this area. The evidence accumulating over the past 10 years about the benefits of physical activity is impressive (see other chapters in this book). Just under one third of all CHD cases and one quarter of strokes could be avoided with appropriate levels of physical activity.

Health benefits of physical activity

In people aged over 45, about a quarter of non insulin dependent diabetes mellitus (NIDDM) and just over half of hip fractures could be prevented with exercise. The report of the US Surgeon General on physical activity for health in 1996[5] sets out many health benefits that can be gained through exercise, which are now widely accepted by experts internationally. These include improved cardiovascular health, better skeletal health, reduced risk of osteoporosis, reduction in both systolic and diastolic blood pressure, reduced incidence of NIDDM, effective weight control, and a reduction in all cause mortality. The role of exercise in raising self esteem, maintaining well-being, managing chronic disease, or in rehabilitation has been well documented and may be particularly important for older people.

The amount of physical activity recommended by experts is 30 minutes of moderate activity on at least 5 days a week. But research shows that six out of 10 men and seven out of 10 women are currently not active enough to get those health benefits. The position is more stark for young people. The recently published National Diet and Nutrition Survey of 4–18 year olds[6] showed that children and young people are extremely inactive – girls are less active than boys, and activity rates decrease with increasing age. About one third of 7–14 year old boys and half of the eldest boys (15–18 year olds) did not meet those Health Development

Agency recommendations for young people to participate in at least moderate intensity activity for one hour per day, and for girls the position was considerably worse. Fifty percent of children walked to school, but only 1–6% cycled and most of these were boys. There is also an emerging trend that children seem to be becoming heavier, even in proportion to their increasing height, largely because they are doing such little activity.

Reasons for inactivity

A recent MORI survey, commissioned by the government as part of the consultation process, looked at why it was that people said they did not exercise. Again, the answers were relatively predictable (Box 1).

Box 1
Factors preventing people from being physically active:

▶ Lack of affordable leisure facilities
▶ Lack of transport (or affordable transport)
▶ Lack of childcare
▶ Lack of time
▶ Concerns about safety and crime

The key question is: what can be done about these issues? People make their own choices about how much or how little to exercise. A 'nagging nanny' state approach is likely to turn people off completely, and would be unlikely to have an impact on the amount of exercise that people do. But there is a clear responsibility to make sure that people are aware of the facts about the health benefits of exercise, and also that they have real genuine opportunities to exercise so that living a healthier life is a real option. That means making it easier for people to be active as part of their daily lives, and building on many of the local programmes that are already making a difference by providing people with more opportunities and raising the levels of activity in local areas. In particular, the focus should be on helping children to have more opportunities for exercise and activity in order for them to get the best start in life.

A co-ordinated approach

The government has taken some of the key initiatives in this area. The Department of Health (DoH) has been working with the Department of Environment and Transport and the Regions (DETR), with the aim of making the environment safer and more attractive for pedestrians and cyclists, and of reducing car-based journeys. The DETR recently published guidance for local authorities on how to encourage walking and putting the pedestrian back at the centre of transport decisions. We have worked very closely with the Department for Education and Employment (DfEE) on the school run; on trying to encourage children to walk or cycle to school, and promoting walking initiatives through the 'safe and sound' challenge (which offered cash prizes to schools that developed innovative walking or cycling schemes). It is clear that the 'walking buses' idea has caught the imagination of many schools and local authorities which shows that pupils, teachers, and those running the schools are thinking seriously about the long-term health benefits of walking. It is that kind of co-operation, both at the national level and at the local level that has the potential to make the biggest difference.

The Department for Culture, Media and Sport has recently published its sports strategy. This recognises the health benefits of increasing participation in sport among the whole population, and for children in particular. The aims are to rebuild sports facilities, create sports colleges to work with primary and secondary schools so as to share good practice and raise standards, and establish 600 school sports co-ordinators to organise coaching, after-school activity and inter-school competitions. The new National Curriculum, effective from September 2000, will set an aim that schools should provide as a minimum two hours per week of curricular or extra curricular activities, with the intention of encouraging a greater emphasis on PE and sports in schools. The Qualifications and Curriculum Authority is leading a project to produce guidance on how schools might best be able to meet this aspiration.

The DoH and DfEE also sponsor the National Healthy School Standards, of which physical activity is one of the core criteria. Health and education partnerships are now in place in all 150 local education authorities to help schools achieve that standard, but clearly we need to go further and there is much more to be done.

As a result of the Diet and Nutrition Survey,[6] we are setting up a working group, drawing together people from across government departments to look specifically at activity and diet in children, to see what more can be done in this key area, and with an aim to develop ideas for proposals to feed into the NHS Plan.

Part of the NSF for CHD includes physical activity as one of the milestones that must be delivered in order to meet the priorities. By April 2001, we expect all NHS bodies working with local authorities to contribute to the delivery of local programmes on increasing physical activity rates. By April 2002, we expect quantitative data on the implementation of these programmes. We have set a goal within the NSF to ensure that patients discharged from hospital following a coronary event are offered exercise programmes as part of their cardiac rehabilitation, and that these sessions are conducted by suitably qualified people. We are in an early stage of implementation of the NSF for CHD but there is the potential to make a difference.

Local initiatives

In many local areas the links at the central government level (as mentioned above) are being picked up and taken even further. Several local health authorities include transport in their health improvement programmes, eg St Helens and Knowsley Health Authority recognises the DETR as a partner in the work they do, and Liverpool Health Authority has also identified improving fitness, social networks and access to employment as part of their health improvement targets. Birmingham's Walk 2000 is a collaboration between Birmingham Health Authority and Birmingham City Council, with support from South Birmingham College.

In 1998, the DETR put out a challenge to all hospitals to lead the change in travel habits. It stated that by the very nature of their work, hospitals should be sending out the right messages to their communities and acting responsibly on health issues. This is the challenge that has been picked up by the NSF for CHD. In due course all NHS facilities will be required to look at their transport plans. Many hospitals are already taking action, eg in Sandwell the hospital transport plans promote pedestrian access to sites, and aim to improve bus services and local bus and cycle networks to the hospitals.

Health professionals at the very local level also have a key role to play. We have seen that general practitioners (GPs) can act as effective levers of change, affecting people's behaviour in a positive way, for example they may help people to give up smoking or alcohol. The GP's potential to extend into other areas of health promotion and prevention of ill health is considerable. Many people pay considerably more attention, understandably, to health messages from their GP than to those from the government or advertising campaigns. Many GPs are keen advocates of health walk programmes, which are important initiatives that often form part of the so called 'exercise on prescription', and this is an initiative the government is keen to promote. It does rely on close liaison between health authorities, local authorities, and primary care teams to offer suitable patients a course of supervised exercise. That might mean patients at risk of heart disease, stroke, diabetes or obesity (these are areas covered in considerable detail in other chapters of this book).

We would be very interested to have your feedback on how you think all this is working, what the potential is, and what the key issues are that will make this work effectively. Clearly, this is going to be only one element and it will not be a panacea. But the evidence from a recent review does indicate that the best exercise referral schemes are very effective and, in the short term, can deliver real increases in activity and therefore health.

Our aim is to improve the quality of these schemes, and to enable GPs to work more effectively with their counterparts in health and local authorities. It is also important that where these schemes and improvements are developed they are sustainable. Many exercise professionals, GPs and academics have assisted in the process of producing a quality assurance framework[7] for GPs to help start those kinds of referral schemes mentioned above, to offer GPs useful contacts and advice on the implications of referral schemes and to highlight the appropriate qualifications of the kind of exercise specialist to whom someone needs to be referred. The aim is to ensure that these programmes are consistent, effective and self-sustaining.

Conclusion

Clearly, we have not yet got all the answers in this area, but there is a huge potential to make a big difference to people's lives. The big question for us is: what will work and what will make a difference? We do not simply want to say we can just put a lot of money into an education campaign to which nobody pays much attention, or which does not deliver real differences in practice. That is why, as part of our approach to evidence based public health, the Health Development Agency has been set up to look at exactly what kind of programmes will make a difference in local areas, deliver real improvements to peoples' health and prevent ill health.

We would be keen to know your views on what you consider would make a difference, what the evidence shows and what it is that we could do to affect a change in this area. There is huge potential. What this is really about is not simply a broad approach to prevention. It is also about tackling the inequalities in ill health and making a real difference to peoples' lives.

Discussion

[Q=question from delegate; YC=Yvette Cooper]

Q Could you elaborate further on the role of exercise for improvements in mental health?

YC The benefits of exercise in mental health can be considerable. We are focusing on the things that make the biggest difference and the links with exercise and mental health are clear. If there are any suggestions in terms of what we ought to do to pick up on that link or what we should do or do differently, I'd be really interested to hear of this.

Q Your comment on the programmes being self-financing raises some concern. How can we prove these programmes work unless funding is made available to look at them long term?

YC How to prove benefits and cost effectiveness is clearly an issue, especially when trying anything new or different, or to obtain funding up front in order to then prove that the funding delivers results. The funding problem for research in the prevention field often occurs because the financial benefits come way down the line. The reason for setting up the Health Development Agency was to try and tackle the deficit that there has been on many of the evidence approaches, eg the difficulties of gathering systematic evidence. It is important to have evidence to justify what we do. We do attempt to pilot things and develop ideas and to have sequel money in order to pilot things to get them up and running so as to gather evidence of their worth. If there are ways in which local areas need to be encouraged to do this, certainly 'Heath Action Zones' have the scope to do exactly that, and to put money into projects and new ideas, in order to prove and to monitor them later on, to show that they are effective. The general feeling is that promotion of physical activity is, in principle, likely to be cost effective. However, it is worth us doing research in order to gather tangible evidence to gain support for expanding these kinds of programmes more broadly.

Q When I helped design a hospital I was told that were no facilities or money for the health service to provide changing rooms, showers or anything else for staff to take exercise on site; it was not part of their remit. I could and do walk to work; but after dark I would not feel safe to walk the streets of Hackney, I would certainly not consider it safe to cycle with heavy traffic, although I am happy to walk or cycle in the countryside. It is easy to say people should cycle or walk to work but I think you need to look at the environment where they work, and what their journeys are, before you can say what is good for their health.

YC The environment is a key issue and one of the reasons why there are a lot of inequalities in this field. If people live in areas of high crime, where they would not want to go out walking or running in the evening, or if financial restraints make it difficult to join convenient gyms, it is clearly much more difficult to exercise or to do so safely. We are attempting to improve environments in general with various schemes, eg 'healthy living centres' which have some potential in reducing barriers to exercising, and applications for projects directed towards low income areas (not only physical buildings) are going into the 'New Opportunities Fund'. These opportunities provide innovative ideas to encourage, for example, walks in a local area or improvements to the environment which might make a difference and make it more realistic for people to be able to exercise.

Q Is there any encouragement for work place physical activity programmes, given the benefits we have seen in the USA, eg reduced absenteeism, increased performance, etc.

YC This is an area in which the NHS as a massive employer needs to do more. We are trying to pick up on some of the issues we talk of as important across the government and implement them through the NHS in a series of different ways which links up with projects such as 'family-friendly' employment. Clearly, access to exercise for staff is an area we should pay more attention to. Within the specifications of NSF CHD there is the scope for trusts and health service employers to take on this responsibility, and the government should encourage this.

We are going to be launching an occupational health strategy shortly. One of the issues apparent from our research into why it is that people find it difficult to exercise and why people don't exercise is their lack of time to do so, given the amount of time they spend at work and other things going on in their lives. Clearly, access to exercise at work has a lot of potential. There are ways to increase activity at work which may not be just about having a gym, eg walking up stairs rather than taking the elevator, walking between office buildings etc. It is actually about promoting ways of making it easier for people to exercise.

Q Exercise and diet are usually talked about collectively. This would suggest an exercise version of a dietician is required and yet no equivalent position exists in the NHS. How long will it be before we see this?

YC The proposal of an exercise equivalent of a dietician is very interesting. This would need to be looked at carefully and if considered appropriate and there was an apparent demand for this role it would then need to be professionally developed. This could be an area people could start working on. The role of an intermediary to advise and support local exercise programmes will be considered as part of the roll out of Quality Assurance Framework.[7]

Q With regard to your comment on outcomes in the NSF: a lot of exercise referral schemes are either based solely in the health authority or reside in the local authority. To try and bring those together and look at the outcomes from a funding perspective is very difficult for the agencies involved with this funding. Please comment.

YC The difficulties of dealing with the pooled funding from local authorities and health authorities is a much-discussed topic. We talk a lot about joined-up government both at national and local levels, and clearly there are all kinds of teething troubles. It is important to improve closer communication between organisations; this makes a huge difference, and has the potential to make far more of a difference. It is something that in many areas is relatively new. Increasingly, there are incentives being put in place and attempts to change budget arrangements, particularly around health and social care. To improve communication across health and local authorities, we need to do more to promote the kind of co-operation we do have. There is some interest, for example, in health improvement plans led by health authorities and community plans led by local authorities. In fact, it is usually the same people involved in the same kinds of issues, and therefore co-ordination and integration for both processes should improve. Everyone is aware that it is an issue and does require attention but I anticipate teething troubles will continue for a while.

References

1   Department of Health. *The NHS Plan – a Plan for Investment, a Plan for Reform.* London: Stationery Office, 2000.
2   Great Britain Independent Inquiry into Inequalities in Health. *Inequalities in Health: the Evidence Presented to the Inquiry into Inequalities in Health, Chaired by Sir Donald Acheson.* London: Stationery Office, 1998.
3   Department of Health. *Saving Lives: our Healthier Nation.* London: Stationery Office, 1999.
4   Department of Health. *National Service Framework for Coronary Heart Disease.* London: DoH, 1999.
5   US Department of Health and Human Services, National Centre for Chronic Disease Prevention and Health Promotion. *Physical Activity and Health – a Report of the Surgeon General.* Atlanta: National Centre for Chronic Disease and Health Promotion, 1996.
6   Office for National Statistics, Social Survey Division. *National Diet and Nutrition Survey – Young People aged 4–18 years (Vol 1).* London: Stationery Office, 2000.
7   Department of Health. *Exercise Referral Systems: a National Quality Assurance Framework.* London: The Stationery Office, 2001.

Address for correspondence: Yvette Cooper MP, Public Health Minister, Richmond House, 79 Whitehall, London SW1A 2NS.

16 The Oliver-Sharpey Lecture
Human performance in health and disease: anatomical and physiological comparisons

Mark Harries

How muscle uses its fuels

Oxygen is an extremely reactive element, and is toxic in high concentrations. Difficulties with its capture from the atmosphere and subsequent distribution have been overcome with the evolution of haemoglobin. When fully saturated, each gram of haemoglobin carries 1.306 ml of oxygen, which is delivered to the mitochondria in muscle via the systemic circulation. Here adenosine tri-phosphate (ATP), the energy currency needed for physiological processes, is formed as the prime product of metabolism of ingested food in all biological systems. Cascades of enzymatic reactions not only harness the forces of oxidation but also serve as a mechanism for disposing of the free radicals that it generates. The rapid provision of ATP for immediate contractile activity is the result of contributions from the muscles' store of phosphocreatine and glycogen. For the first few seconds of maximal exercise, the breakdown of both phosphocreatine and glycogen is responsible for the high rate of ATP production. All-out exercise is therefore instantly possible from rest, providing a vital means of escaping danger.

The biochemical degradation of glycogen can be regarded as a two-phase process. The initial phase takes place without the need for oxygen (anaerobic metabolism). After the first few seconds of maximal exercise, the aerobic degradation of glycogen becomes the main provider of ATP. Power is therefore available using both aerobic and anaerobic systems, each with unique performance advantages and disadvantages (Table 1). The higher the energy demands the greater is the anaerobic component.

The rate of the oxidative processes (aerobic power) is expressed as the product of minute ventilation and the inspired and expired oxygen difference. During peak exercise, sedentary young men typically consume around 40 ml of oxygen per minute per kg of body weight, but are only able to sustain around 60% of this maximum (ie of their $\dot{V}O_2$ max). Fitter

Table 1. Aerobic and anaerobic metabolism.

	Power	Endurance
Mitochondrial (aerobic metabolism)	ATP production is relatively slow	Power is available, without refuelling for days or weeks
Anaerobic metabolism	ATP is generated at 10 times the rate of mitochondrial metabolism	Glucose (glycogen) is the only fuel source and in limited supply <2 hours

individuals reach 60 ml/kg/min but elite endurance athletes may consume in excess of 90 ml of oxygen/kg/min and can sustain this rate for longer. The rise in maximal oxygen consumption seen with training is attributable largely to an increase in oxidative potential of muscle and a greater than 20% improvement in maximal cardiac output. The CO_2 released is twenty times more soluble in water than oxygen. This, and an abundance of the enzyme carbonic anhydrase, ensures that CO_2 can always be absorbed into blood from the tissues and voided from the lungs regardless of the rate at which it is being produced. Thus the critical factor governing aerobic performance is oxygen supply rather than waste disposal.

The relative use of fat or glucose is indicated by the ratio of the volume of carbon dioxide evolved to the volume of oxygen consumed. At the tissue level this is known as the respiratory quotient (RQ), whereas when pulmonary measurements are made it is known as the respiratory exchange ratio (RER). One mole of glucose requires six moles of oxygen for complete oxidation, yielding six moles of carbon dioxide so when glucose is the principal fuel, RER=1 (ie 6/6). Combustion of fat requires a relatively larger volume of oxygen, thus the RER falls below unity. During low intensity exercise RER is around 0.85, indicating that 50% of the energy is derived from fat. But when the work rate is near maximal, almost all the energy comes from glucose. Trained individuals use a relatively higher proportion of fat than the untrained, thereby preserving their glycogen stores.

When the processes of oxygen delivery and extraction reach their limit, more intensive activity is still possible with the anaerobic degradation of glycogen to form lactate. During exercise of moderate to high intensity a substantial amount of the lactate produced is then oxidised for use as an energy substrate by diffusion into neighbouring muscle fibres and by being circulated to the myocardium and the liver. The appearance of lactate in the blood reflects a balance between production and removal.

As exercise intensity increases, production exceeds removal and blood lactate accumulates. A significant rise in blood lactate concentration above resting values can be regarded as the point during exercise beyond which aerobic metabolism can no longer satisfy the demand for ATP.

Changes in blood lactate are used to assess the aerobic fitness of an athlete. For example, the inflection point of the blood lactate exercise-intensity relationship is often described as the 'lactate or anaerobic threshold', though it shows considerable individual variation from 2–6 mmol/l. Others have used a fixed lactate concentration as a reference point, eg 4 mmol/l. and called it the onset of blood lactate accumulation (OBLA). Thereafter, lactate levels rise steeply, curtailing further activity. Oxygen consumption at OBLA is higher in endurance athletes than in sedentary individuals, which again is a feature of their training (Fig 1).

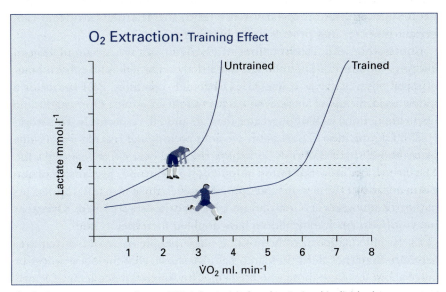

Fig 1. Oxygen consumption at OBLA for trained and untrained individuals.

Disorders of fuel storage

Mammals store their energy as fat or as glycogen, a branched chain polymer of glucose, which aggregates in muscle and the liver. Glycogen is stored close to the mitochondria. Without replenishment it can be consumed in less than two hours, as is demonstrated when comparing muscle biopsy specimens taken before and after exercising to exhaustion. During less intensive exercise, the relative abundance of fat coupled with the need to preserve a substrate for anaerobic power, means that glucose stores are conserved at the expense of fat.

Inborn errors causing impairment of carbohydrate utilisation are relatively rare, but are of great theoretical interest because they provide insights into muscle physiology. They are accompanied by excessive fatigue on exertion. Glycogen accumulates upstream, sometimes causing enlargement of the liver and spleen, affording the term 'glycogen storage diseases'. When myophosphorylase is deficient resulting in type V glycogen storage disease (McArdle's syndrome), only blood glucose is available for glycolysis and so, although some anaerobic power is available, intensive exercise is curtailed. But a deficiency of phospho-fructokinase (Tarui's disease, type VII disease) results in complete inability to utilise glucose.[1] Fat then becomes the only source of fuel, reflected in the low respiratory exchange ratio, and physical activity is severely impaired (Fig 2). However, during sustained, low intensity exercise, mobilisation of fatty acids (and, in McArdle's syndrome, of hepatic glucose) may provide a second wind.

Contrasting with abnormalities of glycogen storage, accumulation of excessive amounts of fat, although not strictly regarded as an inborn error of metabolism as far as is known, is extremely common. BMI kg/m^2, is a widely used means of measuring excess weight in adults. Overweight and obese are defined as BMI of greater than 25 and 30, respectively. The World Health Organisation classification provides an index of risk of co-morbidity places those with a BMI over 30 at high risk, and over 40, at very high risk. The British are now the fattest population in Europe, just ahead of the Germans, with 17% of male and 20% of female adults with a BMI in excess of 30.[2] Twenty years ago, only around 7% of Britons were obese. Over that time too, German schoolchildren have doubled their obesity rate.

The problem appears to be not that obese people eat a lot but that they eat more than they need. Research has also shown that the obese fidget or move about less than those who are lean. The American Academy of Sports Medicine has stressed the crucial role of physical activity in maintaining aerobic fitness and controlling weight:[3] 'At least 20–60 min of continuous or intermittent aerobic activity should be taken 3–5 days per week'. Yet the number of 10–13 year-olds taking regular physical exercise at school is falling. What is more, the sale of school playing fields has caused a decline in the numbers participating in team sports.

Calorie restriction without a concomitant increase in physical activity is seldom successful in achieving substantial weight loss, but dietary considerations are important none-the-less. During their arduous training course it has been estimated that the average Royal Marine will require a daily intake of more than 7,000 kcal simply to maintain body weight,

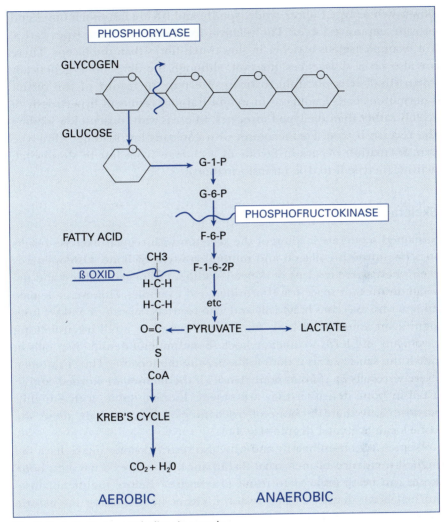

Fig 2. Carbohydrate metabolism in muscle.

whereas some sedentary individuals may gain weight on less than 1,500 kcal. Ideally up to 60% of the calories consumed should be in the form of complex carbohydrate such as potatoes or pasta, with less than 30% fat.[4] The bulk should be eaten at breakfast and in the early part of the day with only a carbohydrate snack taken before retiring.

Responses of muscle to exercise

Human limb muscle contains only three myosin-heavy-chain isoforms: I, IIa, and IIb. Activities which predominantly require endurance utilise slow-twitch or type I fibres, while type IIa and IIb are fast-twitch fibres and provide explosive force.[5] The relative distribution of these types varies. For example, soleus is richer in slow-twitch fibres than the biceps. There are also racial differences, however, although the fibre mix is genetically controlled, it is possible to train one type in favour of the other. Intermittent high loading as in weight training results in hypertrophy of type II rather than the type I myocytes, whereas with constant low loading the reverse is true. Furthermore, with constant low loading, fibre-type transformation occurs in favour of a change from fast to slow-twitch activity, (ie type II to type I transformation).

Skeletal responses to exercise

Sustained moderate loading of the skeleton with regular exercise results in a rise in both collagen and mineral content of bone. Osteopenia is seen where there is a lack of skeletal loading. Prolonged bed rest and the weightlessness of space travel provide good examples. However, a female athlete who exercises habitually and who restricts her calorie intake, loses significant amounts of body fat. This is linked to a fall in circulating oestrogen and leads to amenorrhoea. Bone mineral density then falls in much the same way as it does following the menopause. Thus in women exercise results in a rise in bone density if the menses are normal, and in a fall in bone density if they are absent. Lumbar spine, with a higher turnover rate than the bone of trochanter or femoral shaft, shows the bone loss to a greater degree (Fig 3).[6]

Women who train heavily and who also restrict calorie intake have the highest incidence of menstrual disturbance. In anorexia nervosa, bone losses can be so great as to result in fracture.[7] Before the menopause, normal bone density can be restored either by increasing the calorie intake or with hormone replacement therapy and preferably, with both.[8] But if menses are absent for more than six months, normal bone density may never be fully restored.

Excessive repetitive skeletal loading can also give rise to breakdown of the underlying bone structure, and then spontaneous fracture (stress fracture). Often the fracture line is not visible on the X-ray, but shows up on nuclear scanning due to increased surrounding osteoblastic activity. CT-scanning of the hot spot best reveals the fracture site.

Cardiac responses to exercise

Sustained pressure loading of the left ventricle in hypertension gives rise to hypertrophy, whereas the constant volume loading of failure leads to

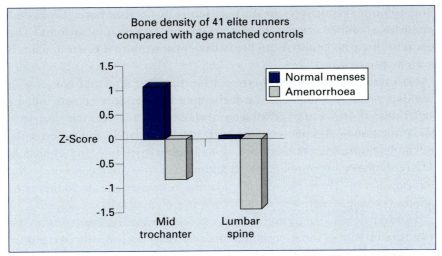

Fig 3. Skeletal responses to exercise. (Reproduced from ref [6] with permission).

dilatation. The athlete's heart is subjected to both pressure and volume loading, but of limited duration only (usually less than 6 hours per day). So although both hypertrophy and dilatation of the ventricle are seen in varying degrees (Fig 4), the change is seldom pathological. For example, wall thickness rarely measures more than 16 mm in diastole, with chamber diameter more than 60 mm in diastole, compared with <11mm

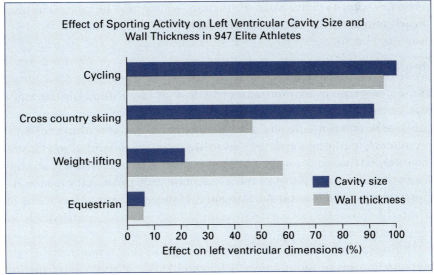

Fig 4. Cardiac adaptations to exercise. (Reproduced from ref [9] with permission).

and <55mm respectively in normal subjects. Cyclists have the largest recorded chamber size overall and rowers the thickest myocardium.[9] The greatest disparity between the two, where hypertrophy is predominant, is seen in weight lifters.

An increase in stroke volume and ejection fraction that comes with training means that adequate cardiac output can be achieved with a lower heart rate. In highly trained athletes, the ECG recorded during sleep may show rates below 20 bpm with sino-atrial block. Dilatation and hypertrophy of the left ventricle coupled with sinus bradyarrhythmias and abnormal ECG complexes are commonly seen and have been termed collectively 'the athlete's heart'. These changes are adaptive responses, cardiac dimensions and ECG changes regress towards normal as soon as activity is reduced.

Sudden death occurring during exercise is a rare event. Amongst young adults, the most common predisposing factor is hypertrophic obstructive cardiomyopathy (HOCM) in which left ventricular wall thickness ranges up to 60 mm (mean 22 mm). The hypertrophy is patchy in distribution being greatest in the septum (septum/wall thickness exceeding 1.5/1). The septal wall encroaches onto the outflow tract in systole obstructing blood flow and causing syncope during exercise. Prevalence is less than one per thousand. Hypertrophic and familial dilated cardiomyopathies, including those involving the right ventricle, have approximately one tenth the incidence of HOCM. Most of these conditions have now been traced to specific genetic mutations.[10] In older athletes, death in the course of physical exertion is more commonly associated with underlying coronary artery disease. Invariably, the terminal event is ventricular fibrillation, which may be preceded by a broad complex tachy-arrhythmia (Fig 5).

Respiratory responses to exercise

During exercise, in extreme cases, the flow of blood through the lungs may exceed 50 l/min, whilst airflow can approach 300 l/min. Blood and air are separated only by the thickness of the alveolar-capillary membrane, and yet pulmonary haemorrhage is rare. Mixing is so efficient that the erythrocytes emerge fully saturated with oxygen even at high levels of exertion, leading to the assumption that pulmonary factors do not normally limit aerobic performance. However recent observations of arterial hypoxaemia occurring during all-out exercise, particularly in female athletes, refute this.[11]

During maximal sustained exercise, ventilation closely matches the rate of oxygen consumption. Minute ventilation (MV) is largely governed by the diameter of the central airways, but less so by the bronchioles because

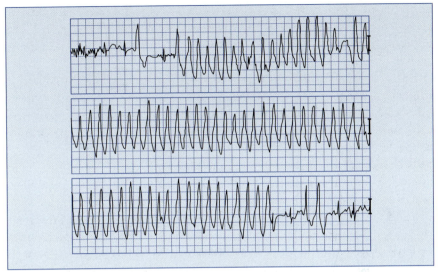

Fig 5. Arrhythmia due to right ventricular cardiomyopathy.

there are many more of them giving rise to a larger cross-sectional area. Expiratory airflow is maximal when the bronchi are at their widest (ie at full inspiration) and lowest towards residual volume as the airways narrow. Change in airflow rate throughout the entire respiratory cycle is depicted by the maximal effort flow-volume loop, which describes the envelope within which all respiratory efforts are contained (Fig 6). During sustained maximal exercise, flow rate limitation occurs during expiration but never on inspiration. Minute ventilation can be estimated by converting average forced expiratory flow (FEF 75-25 l/s) to l/min, and dividing by two, since expiration occupies only about half of the respiratory cycle (MV l/min) $\approx$ (FEF 75–25 l/s) $\times$ 30 (Fig 6).

Given minute ventilation, the equation can be worked backwards to calculate average expiratory flow during exercise. When plotted on the expiratory portion of the maximum effort flow-volume loop, this value indicates at what percentage of vital capacity breathing is taking place. Most athletes breathe at around 50% of their vital capacity during sustained vigorous exercise, rising to over 80% when asked to breathe as vigorously as possible for ten seconds (maximum voluntary ventilation, MVV). In severe obstructive airways disease, airflow is low throughout all of expiration. To achieve adequate ventilation, sufferers are obliged to breathe very close to total lung capacity,[12] which they can manage only by chronically loading their respiratory muscles. Biopsy samples taken from the diaphragm of these individuals show exactly what might be expected, with an excess of type I and a reduction in the number of type II fibres.[13]

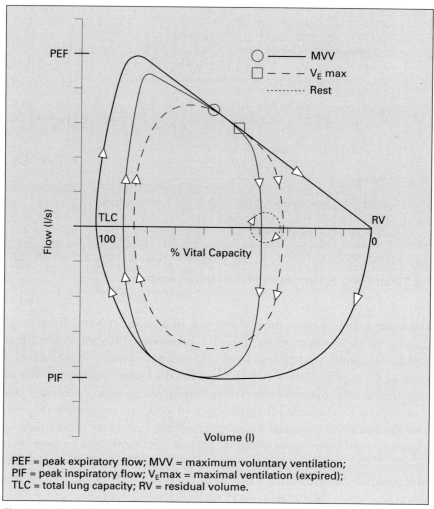

Fig 6. Maximal effort flow-volume loop.

References

1   Haller R, Lewis S. Glucose-induced exertional fatigue in muscle phosphofructokinase deficiency. *N Engl J Med* 1991; **324**: 364–9.
2   Gleick E. Land of the fat. *Time magazine* 1999; **17**: 70–80.
3   Pollock ML, Gorsser GA, Butcher JD. The recommended quantity and quality of exercise for developing and maintaining cardiorespiratory and muscular fitness in healthy adults. *Med Sci Sports Exerc* 1998; **30**: 975–91.
4   Williams C. Nutrition. In: Harries M, Williams D, Stanish W, Micheli L (eds). *Oxford Textbook of Sports Medicine (2e)*. Oxford: Oxford University Press, 1998.
5   Larsson L, Moss RL. Maximum velocity of shortening in relation to myosin isoform composition in single fibres from human skeletal muscles. *J Physiol (Lond)* 1993; **472**: 595–614.

6 Wilson J, Reeve J, Harris MG. Determinants of bone mineral density in female athletes. *Bone* 1994; **15**: 450.

7 Drinkwater BL, Nilson K, Chesnut CH, *et al.* Bone mineral content of amenorrheic and eumenorrheic athletes. *N Eng J Med* 1984; **311**: 277–81.

8 Gibson L, Mitchell A, Reeve J, Harries M. Treatment of reduced bone mineral density in athletic amenorrhoea: a pilot study. *Osteoporosis Int* 1999; **10**: 284–9.

9 Spirito P, *et al.* Morphology of the 'athlete's heart' assessed by echo-cardiography in 947 elite athletes representing 27 sports. *Am J Cardiol* 1994; **74**: 802–6.

10 Fatkin D, *et al.* Missense mutations in the rod domain of the lamin A/C gene as causes of dilated cardiomyopathy and am-system disease. *N Eng J Med* 1999; **341** No 23: 1715–24.

11 Harmes C, McLaran S, Nickele G, *et al.* Exercise-induced arterial hypoxaemia in healthy young women. *J Physiol (Lond)* 1998; **507**: 619–28.

12 Babb T. Mechanical ventilatory constraints in ageing, lung disease, and obesity: perspectives and a brief review. *Med Sci Sports Exerc* 1999; **31**: S12–22.

13 Levine S, Kaiser L, Leferovich M, Tikunov B. Cellular adaptations in the diaphragm in chronic obstructive pulmonary disease. *N Eng J Med* 1997; **337**: 1799–806.